I0122764

SELF-CARE IN HEALTHCARE

SELF-CARE
IN HEALTHCARE

CARING for Yourself as You Care for Others

DEBORAH S. HOWELL

Published by Victory in Action LLC, Las Vegas, Nevada
© 2018 by Deborah S. Howell
Printed in the United States of America

All rights reserved. No part of this publication may be reproduced or transmitted in any form or by any means, electronic or mechanical, including photocopying, recording, or by any information storage and retrieval system, without the prior written permission from the publisher or the author. Contact the publisher for information on foreign rights.

ISBN: 978-0-9829284-6-2 (paperback)
         978-0-9829284-0-0 (ebook)

Cover and Interior Design by Carolyn Sheltraw
www.csheltraw.com

Victory in Action image created by Michelle K. Ponimoi

Photos of Deborah Howell (back cover) taken by Michael Gordon

VICTORY IN ACTION®

VICTORY IN ACTION® and its image is a registered trademark owned by Deborah Howell

Disclaimer: The content in this book is NOT INTENDED as medical advice or to diagnose, treat, cure, or prevent any medical or mental condition. It is NOT in any way intended as a substitute for medical or psychological counseling. The suggestions, ideas, and exercises shared in this book have been helpful to me, but may not have the same benefit for you. You should consult with a licensed physician for anything that relates to your overall health, which includes appropriate medical treatment or any anticipated/planned changes to your diet or exercise routine.

♾ The paper used in this publication meets the minimum requirements of the American National Standard for Information sciences—Permanence of Paper for Printed Library Materials, ANSI Z39.48-1992.

www.victoryinaction.com

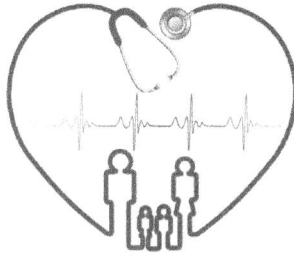

DEDICATION

It is with Gratitude and Inspiration for each day of my life that I dedicate this book to YOU, who are ready to live your best life possible. Life offers opportunities and challenges for personal growth, self-reflection, and enlightenment. I desire that this book be a trustworthy resource to guide you to deeper understanding, appreciation, and acceptance of your life experiences. Be inspired and empowered to rise in faith and strength. Engage in self-leadership recognizing your life matters and your life has purpose. May this book awaken insight, conscientiousness, and wisdom forever impacting your life and future generations to come.

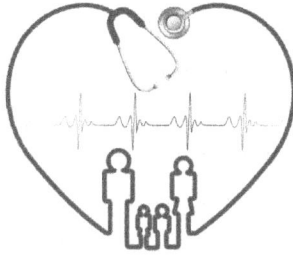

ACKNOWLEDGMENTS

Special thank you to my beautiful family and friends for your love and faith in me. You helped to lift and move me forward every time you checked-in with me to find out if my book was "done yet" and offered me words of encouragement.

An extra special thank you to my husband for your patience with my long hours at work and for preparing the most delicious gourmet meals that have helped sustain my daily efforts!

Sincere thank you to my mom and daughter Erika for generously giving your time and thoughtful attention to help me edit this book. I am so grateful for your love and support throughout this process.

A very special thank you to my friend Fran, whose heart and tenacity inspired me from the first day we met. You have been a pillar of wisdom and strength, a sounding board, and a cheerleader encouraging me to step up and out into the world to share my heart and passion. Your life is a true testament to what dedication and commitment means when standing in your truth, going above and beyond what has been seemingly impossible. You are simply amazing! I am ever grateful for our connection!

A warm thank you to my graphic designer. You have helped me bring my ideas to life. You are extremely talented, insightful, and trustworthy. I am truly grateful for the opportunity to work with you!

I would like to express my sincere appreciation for all of you who serve in our healthcare system. It is a noble and gratifying service with many challenges. Your perspective on caring for yourself matters. I invite you to explore what brings meaning and purpose to your life. Take time to care for yourself as you continue the great work and experience the joy of caring for others.

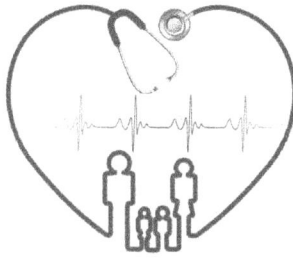

TABLE OF CONTENTS

"In order to change an existing paradigm
you do not struggle to try and change the
problematic model. You create a new model
and make the old one obsolete."

~ R. Buckminster Fuller

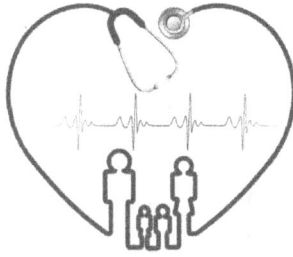

PREFACE:
THE BUSINESS
OF LIVING WELL

PERSONAL RESPONSIBILITY:
COMMITMENT AND DISCIPLINE TO SELF-LEADERSHIP

CHOOSING TO CULTIVATE GOOD
HEALTH ON A DAILY BASIS:
PLAN, PREPARE, PRACTICE

MAKING YOUR HEALTH A TOP PRIORITY:
DECISION, CORE VALUES, COMMUNITY

It is an honor and privilege to share with you what I truly feel and have experienced is the most viable and practical way we can restructure our healthcare system.

I am proposing a way forward through self-care management as a sustainable model that can work for all of us when we recognize and value the preciousness and possibilities of the life we have been granted and choose to live our best life possible.

I offer thoughts, insights, and experiences, and touch on evidenced based findings to help support, guide, and expand individual and collective views of effective options for self-care management. I hope that this information will support your personal inquiry and pursuits and support the initiation and ongoing personal care and quality of life conversations with your families, patients, clients, organizations.

The cultivation of this book stems from personal and professional frustration that led me to seek answers and support for what I have struggled with for a long time. One would think that self-care is a natural and easy thing to do and maintain, however, most of us are running on empty and on autopilot. We are struggling with overcare, not paying attention, or frankly not caring until we are halted in our tracks by injury, illness, or crisis. Habits tend to run the show until the show can no longer go on. Self-care management is a relatively simple solution yet it has its challenges. The necessity for self-care is truly about the inner work, identifying the beliefs, influences, perspectives, and motivations that drive our behaviors.

I am deeply passionate about this topic for my own personal well-being and for the patients and people around me that I love and work with everyday. I have learned through my experiences that there are 3 key factors for an effective and sustainable self-care management program. These are commitment, consistency, and community.

- *Is your health a top priority?*
- *Do you feel empowered and motivated towards living a happy and healthy life?*
- *What are you cultivating on a daily basis with your choices, habits, and behaviors?*
- *How are you caring for yourself?*

My intention for this topic of self-care is to return us to caring for humanity, to shed light on how we can share in effectively and compassionately caring for one another as we take better care in our own lives. Rising out of frustration and appreciation, I believe that aligning our core values from all perspectives can help us to join in collaboration of our efforts to put the care back into health care. I am deeply passionate about this matter after personally experiencing for a period of time, depletion and discouragement as both a patient and therapy practitioner. We all have expectations and perspectives of how we want to feel, be treated and at the end of the day know that our efforts have made a difference and our lives matter.

- *As a healthcare provider or caregiver, how do you feel about the quality of care you provide your patients? How well do you care for yourself?*
- *As a client or as the patient, how do you feel about the quality of care you are receiving from your healthcare provider? What responsibility do you have in better caring for yourself?*

This book proposes that we explore how we define care, manage care, deliver care, experience care, and MODEL care which also include the processes and politics around care. The desired outcome is to introduce a paradigm shift to a more engaged, transparent, and collaborative model to include an emphasis on self-care. The fundamental values of heart centered and patient centered care have been diluted and slowly drifted over time to an automated, mechanical, desensitized, detached, and at times a seemingly dehumanized health care delivery system.

From my perspective covering over two decades, what has developed is an infiltration of greed and distrust resulting in propagating self-serving initiatives that omit, manipulate, adjust and justify to meet one's own agenda. Competition amongst insurance carriers, health care institutions, practitioners, alongside the misuse, abuse, fraud, manipulation and less than optimal self-care behaviors have all contributed to a massive system disconnect and breakdown. This disconnect has led to a system that reasons and makes decisions referred to as cost-effective, however, I believe this is nothing more than an excuse to "legitimately" hold back or hold off on previously valued provisions as we continue to expect and mandate more without full appreciation or consideration of long-term consequences to the quality of our human experiences and potential. The subtle dilution over the years has been working behind the scenes yet now, can be witnessed and experienced at every level of the system. I have witnessed the anguish and pain of people who have been denied coverage and services that they could benefit from because they did not meet criteria to qualify for funding of the service or product. We are all subject to the same forces in life, some to a greater or lesser degree, and we cannot anticipate what we may face and subsequently need over the course of our lifespan.

- *How can we collaborate to better care for each other in this health care model and get ourselves back on track to recognizing the things that really matter?*

I am truly grateful for my experiences as a physical therapist. This profession has offered the most rewarding and enlightening experiences beyond what I could have ever imagined and to be able to adequately convey in words. I have had the opportunity to serve in various roles within the healthcare infrastructure as a physical therapist, admissions liaison, and case manager. I have had specialized training in women's and men's health, neuro and oncology rehabilitation, and have worked in a variety of settings which include home health care, out-patient and private practice, acute care, skilled care, and acute and long-term inpatient rehabilitation. From these experiences, I have gained insight and understanding to recognize and appreciate that health care is a business. What concerns me with this knowledge is that I have seen a shift in priorities and a widening gap in communication as a result of this health care business detaching true "care" from the original focus of health care which is impacting the quality of health care delivery and utility as we experience it today. My deeper concern with this reality explores this issue on a more personal level for we are all subject to needing and utilizing resources from this system at various points in our lives.

We have in essence an interpersonal relationship built around a model which has many different access, touch, and reference points offering up many different perspectives and subsequent challenges. As a consumer, my question for you both the patient and the practitioner is whether you have considered and reflected upon what is your personal responsibility and expectation with respect to this business model which we all need to have access to yet may have potential for limited or denied access based on known and unknown criteria.

Health care is everyone's business and responsibility, however, what I have observed and experienced is a huge disconnect in our system today at every level. We have wandered so far off the central path of caring and genuine heartfelt concern for the well-being of humanity. Much of what we see is automated and mechanical, simply out of touch. Many people have lost their enthusiasm, feel unappreciated, burnt out, and have lost trust, or feel entitled without any sense of personal responsibility or accountability. At the micro-level, referring to direct patient care, respective processes and agendas are often on parallel paths. Instead of an integrative and collaborative model, we are experiencing huge gaps in communication to include the fear of misinterpretation, fraud, abuse, and misuse.

- *Where does Self-Care fit in?*

Self-care is a daily act of caring for oneself which include self-awareness, self-support, and self-influence. Blaming, shaming, and tasking someone else with up to 100% of the responsibility for personal health and self-care primarily through corrective measures (medications, surgeries, therapies, etc.) for what is essentially our individual responsibility keep us away from where we truly want to be and how we truly want to feel.

- *How do you typically feel throughout the day, and at the end of your day?*
- *Are you energized and inspired by your experiences?*
- *How honest are you about recognizing your part in achieving and sustaining good health, in being and living well?*

At any point in time, we have an opportunity to become more aware, make a new or different decision, choose to improve on a situation, and take action in the direction of where we want to go or how we want to feel.

Self-care is EVERYONE's responsibility. It is a collective and collaborative distribution of care that offers self-sustaining and self-engaging returns, and is collectively rewarding. Presently, we are spread thin due to lack of nourishing and nurturing self-care practices.

Some may think that self-care is a nice "idea" however, as I have observed through close and personal interaction with patients is that self-care is essential as a way forward to improving the quality of our lives and the quality of our health care delivery system. It is a moment-to-moment awareness and presence that provides us vital information, the truth of the moment when we learn to actively listen. We are struggling to perform daily caring tasks because we are misaligned with what we say we want compared to what we are actually doing to support our desires.

We are in conflict both externally and internally with an organic process called change. We are challenged with seeking ways to standardized care within the confines of semi-rigid to rigid processes and policies that miss the mark on validating the true "meaning" of what we desire to achieve by this action or inaction. This reference is to outcomes that offer meaningful rewards or consequences. For what I have experienced and possibly you can relate, it feels like there are more undesirable consequences that are taking a toll on our lives and livelihood.

> Adapting to change and resiliency is inherent to Mother Nature. That is how we grow and evolve... becoming better, wiser, faster, and stronger.

Proper self-care organically has a way of engaging and supplying us the fuel to support our greatest and truest desires. Self-care should be encouraged to not feel like "work." It can be simple, practical, and effective with small yet meaningful decisions we make that support a body that desires to thrive in a healthy environment both internally and externally. To talk about caring and the actual demonstration of caring are oftentimes at opposite ends of the spectrum. The current automation of delivering care is not satisfying for any of us. When we interact with one another there is an exchange happening. We exchange information on both a verbal and non-verbal level. When we care for ourselves, we are better able to sustain caring for others from a natural place of overflow instead of the typical overwhelm. I know this for myself and as I observe healthcare providers, patients, and families, I see an awful lot of burdened and distressed appearances that I honestly feel could be much different if we knew how to do different. Not just the knowledge of doing different but the motivation that naturally self-perpetuates and reinforces because the outcome contains its own rewards.

As we move through our day, we take on more than we realize...the wounds, fears, traumas and dramas subtly work their way into our energy fields and into our cells affecting our well-being. Consistently caring for ourselves is a requirement to effectively care for others. Developing our capacity and resiliency helps us to sustain good health, a positive attitude, the ability to critically think and listen empathically. We are so busy doing what we are trained to do or feel obligated to do that we have lost sight of why we are doing it and lost the enthusiasm and compassion to support our daily efforts. We are not feeling inspired and fulfilled by the care we are providing others and find little or no time to care for ourselves.

> The physician who is talking about health and prescribing medications to improve health yet engages in unhealthy behaviors could be considered hypocritical, as well as the patient who expects the doctor or therapist to "fix" them could be considered irresponsible.

Medical guidance in health care is delivered not only through direct means, but is also indirectly communicated through observation and felt sense of genuine compassion and concern. Whether we are at a regular doctor visit or we are sick and suffering, our reference for information, support, and hope often becomes the person or persons we meet entrusted to care for us and to guide us, more so when we are alone or needing encouragement.

Most of us would agree that good health and a sense of well-being is cultivated through daily self-care practices. Extensive research has validated that regular physical activity can reduce the incidence and prevalence of many chronic diseases. A national survey on personal exercise habits and counseling practices of primary care physicians revealed that Americans look to their physicians as their primary source of information regarding healthy lifestyle decisions and those physicians who regularly perform aerobic exercise and / or strength training were more likely to talk to their patients on the benefits of these exercises.[1] The survey also identified that the factors of inadequate time, knowledge, or experience regarding exercise were the most common barriers to physicians not engaging in healthy lifestyle discussions. This information supports the physician and practitioner model of care that I am an advocate for as an effective behavioral strategy for improving dialogue, education, and personal example for better engagement and encouragement of self-care strategies and management.

Directing efforts on self-management can help improve outcomes for chronic pain care. A relevant article on the American Pain Society's web site[2] highlighted the National Pain Strategy focus on patient education and self-management as being a vital path to improving the treatment of chronic pain and reducing pain-related disability. The article mentioned that the Institute of Medicine estimated that 100 million Americans are dealing with persistent or chronic pain and for people less than 45 years old, back pain was the leading cause of disability. Self-management programs are interventions that teach people how to help themselves become more active and manage their symptoms. These programs also help to reduce the stigma, frustration, and minimize depression and other accompanying mood disorders.

"Self-Management is good medicine."

~Albert Bandura

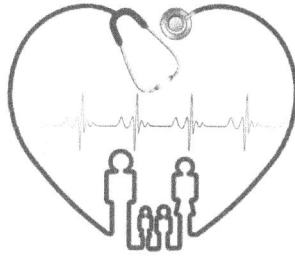

CHAPTER 1

ACT ON YOUR HEALTH

YOUR LIFE MATTERS
Live Up to Your Greatest Potential!

In each of our lives, let us achieve a sense of inner peace and purpose—understanding and acceptance of our own personal truths, and recognizing that our life's inherent purpose extends beyond our individual lives. May we learn to love one another with an Agape kind of love that reaches deeply inside without the need for words or special deeds. May we begin to practice the kind of presence that embodies a compassionate and gentle spirit, enabling us to openly acknowledge and appreciate the vulnerability of man's heart and soul, and recognize the authenticity of genuine human connection for healing, restoration, and unity.

It is my passion and intention to provide incentives and examples to empower and encourage you...offer you hope, inspiration, and insight to help you maximize on the life you have been given. I desire to assist you in making sense of your life and to expand your view of what is possible. I hope to increase your awareness on all that is available to you to experience when you open your eyes, mind, and heart to all that is inherently present and to all that can possibly be.

The use of "real life" depictions and "true life" situations is to motivate you to live proactively with a sense of hope and empowerment, and to take personal responsibility for your life. Allow me to assist you in finding the courage to rebuild a healthy, loving foundation—to develop a root system of love, faith, and gratitude that will nurture and nourish you as it works its way outward through you...creating a ripple effect into the masses that are hungry for loving human kindness.

My experiences in the military and in health care have taught me a great deal about life and about people and relationships. I continue to learn about human behavior, human needs and desires, and the true meaning of humanity. All of our lives have value and everyone has the right to be treated with dignity, respect, competent and compassionate care.

> You can choose to live an Inspired life… to see the beauty, strength, and tenderness in every heart you are privileged to connect with.

- *How do you define success?*
- *What does it mean to you to be successful?*
- *What does success feel or look like to you?*
- *Is success a point of destination you are striving to reach?*

Life is an ongoing process of living, learning, and growing in the moment; relating to the moment with ease or resistance. We can choose to capture, dismiss, or remain oblivious to the messages and teachings from the experiences in our daily lives—experiences that are represented as small, cumulative moments. Life offers a continuum and a medium—a journey and an opportunity—allowing us to learn, adapt, modify, embrace, recognize, grow, prosper, restore, and heal. I believe the journey intends for our success and extends a purposeful path lined with teach-ings and lessons for our navigation. There is inherent meaning built into life experiences; merit and purpose for us all to dis-cover. Many of us fail to recognize this because we get caught-up, side-tracked, derailed — feeling "stuck" due to life's traumas and dramas occurring in our daily lives.

- *How do we make sense of it all?*
- *How do we gain insight and wisdom from our struggles?*
- *How do we get over the hurdles, through the breakups and the breakdowns, and survive the pitfalls?*
- *How are we to rise out of discouragement and despair as a result of our hurts, injuries, and scars?*
- *How do we find our way after traumatic experiences have left us feeling violated, ill-equipped, disabled, disillusioned, depressed, disheartened, or destroyed?*

I am eager and excited to expose you to practical insights and perspectives of the world, a world of opportunity, hope, and enlight-ened living. I ask you to open your heart and all your senses as you read through this book. You will notice that I utilize "we" in much of the material to encourage a collective consciousness and involve-ment; to realize this information applies to all of us and influences the collective processing of life's experiences and challenges. I will refer to "you" as a means to assist you, the reader, in gaining a more personal appreciation for how the information can directly affect and impact your life. I share with you information to facilitate an increase in your sense of self-worth and to validate your being; to teach you how to nourish your mind, body, and spirit with healthier choices, positive influences, and positive, loving, and empower-ing self-talk . . . raising consciousness and inspiring you to connect to a source of greatness that resides within you. My intention and desire is to provide you with a valuable, enlightening resource that presents itself as a friend, confidant, and mentor to assist, support, and guide you through your day-to-day experiences, challenges, interactions, and decisions.

May your hope and faith be realized and forever restored. Rise with strength and courage! Know that you are loved, supported, and valued. Recognize your heart's ability and resiliency to overcome grief, despair, disappointment, and trauma — allowing you to experience love, forgiveness, and healing. Be empowered to dream and to proactively navigate on your intended path to success, making the necessary changes and adjustments along the way. Tap into a sense of personal victory through the discovery of your inherent core value and ultimately connecting with your life's meaning and purpose.

PERSONAL INVITATION TO ACT ON YOUR HEALTH

Invitation to Act On Your Health!

My personal mission is to make a positive impact on global health starting with YOU, the consumer — the health professional, the parent, the student, the employer, the employee, the self-employed, all of you who desire information, support, and an opportunity to create positive change in your life. I hope to empower YOU, the individual, with information and resources — to promote awareness and facilitate social and behavioral change — to inspire personal transformation.

- *What can we do individually and collectively to improve the quality of our lives and the quality of our healthcare?*

The quality of our health and healthcare is immediate and central to our livelihood and our quality of life. We are all impacted by health in some aspect where we want to look good and feel good and be treated with competent care while preserving dignity and respect.

STRESS and poor nutritional choices directly contribute to the onset and exacerbation of chronic illnesses such as cancer, heart disease, diabetes, obesity, depression, and many other debilitating conditions. Most people are taken by complete surprise when the seemingly sudden onset of illness strikes. Act On Your Health is a call for immediate and decisive action; a call for each of you to recognize your personal value; a call for collective consciousness to facilitate a massive shift individually and globally with regard to awareness, attitudes, and behaviors affecting the state of our health, economy, and overall well-being today. What would it mean to you, your family, our society, our health care system, etc., if we could decrease the incidence of chronic illnesses? The manifestation of most illnesses is significantly influenced by lifestyle, based on daily choices and rooted in attitudes and behaviors learned from childhood.

When crisis strikes a family, everyone is shocked, saddened, and all of a sudden, life has changed without warning. So many questions are asked, many without a definitive answer. Throughout the course of my career, I've witnessed the devastating and life-altering effects of chronic illness. Can you imagine how one's life is changed when a leg is amputated because of an ongoing infection due to circulation problems from diabetes—a sudden heart attack happens requiring the use of a ventilator (breathing machine)—a stroke occurs that weakens or paralyzes the body—an accident happens resulting in a head injury or spinal cord injury where one has to learn how to eat, talk, and walk again.

My twenty-three years as a physical therapist have opened my eyes, heart, and mind to renewed possibilities for a healthier, happier future for millions of lives. It has been an honor and privilege for me to assist people to regain their health and their livelihood; to be an integral part of the recovery – rehabilitative process for thousands of patients and their families. My personal and professional experiences have lead me to create services that educate, inspire, and motivate people of all ages, encouraging the necessary shift in personal beliefs and behaviors. It is my sincere desire to share my knowledge and experiences with you, in hopes of sparing you and your family the pain and suffering of life-altering debility and the heartache of losing loved ones unexpectedly. This book offers you health information and resources. As you read, may you discover new insights and opportunities that will forever change your life!

Top 10 Leading Causes of Death[1]:

1. Heart Disease
2. Cancer
3. Chronic Lower Respiratory Disease
4. Accidents (Unintentional Injury)
5. Stroke
6. Alzheimer's Disease
7. Diabetes
8. Influenza & Pneumonia
9. Kidney Disease
10. Suicide

Leading Causes of Death and Disability in the United States

These are the Most Common, Costly, and Preventable:

Heart Disease

Stroke

Cancer

Type 2 Diabetes

Obesity

Arthritis

As of 2012:

Fifty-percent of all adults had one or more chronic health condition
= 117 million people
1 out of 4 Adults had two or more of these chronic conditions.

Heart Disease and Cancer combined accounted for nearly 48% of all deaths in 2014.

Diabetes is the leading cause of kidney failure, lower-limb amputations (not from injury), and blindness among adults.

Obesity is a major health concern. From 2011-2014, more than one-third of adults were considered obese. About one out of six youths between ages 2–19 years of age were identified as being obese.

Arthritis is the most common cause of disability.

Overview from the Center for Disease Control and Prevention Website[2]

CHRONIC HEALTH CONDITIONS ARE COSTLY!

In 2010, 86% of all Health Care spending was for people with one or more chronic medical conditions!

$316.1 billion: Total annual costs Cardiovascular Disease in 2012-2013.
$157 billion: Cancer Care costs in 2010
$245 billion: Total estimated costs of Diabetes in 2012.
$147 billion: Estimated Medical costs linked to obesity in 2008.
$128 billion: Total costs of Arthritis and related conditions in 2003.

HEALTH RISK BEHAVIORS THAT CAUSE CHRONIC DISEASES

Health risk behaviors are considered unhealthy behaviors that cause much of the illness, suffering, and early death attributed to chronic diseases. **These health risk behaviors are in your control to change!**

Center for Disease Control (CDC) highlights four of these health risk behaviors:

- Lack of Exercise or Physical Activity
- Poor Nutrition
- Smoking – Tobacco use
- Excessive Alcohol consumption

IMPORTANT NOTICE:
Centers For Disease Control (CDC) and Prevention information is subject to change and periodic updates. Please check for updates and access additional information on Chronic Diseases on the CDC Website:
https://www.cdc.gov/chronicdisease/overview/index.htm

Overview from the Center for Disease Control and Prevention Website[2]

CONVENIENCE IS KILLING US
Get Healthy — Your Body Is Talking

- *What is the true cost of convenience?*
- *What do we see as a result of great marketing and deceptive advertising?*

Look around in your own lives. Those of us in health care can appreciate that medications and procedures have extended lives, but *what can be said about the details of quality of life?* More and more people are starting at a younger age to rely on medication for physical and/or mental stability, are on a transplant list waiting for a vital organ, rely on dialysis for survival, and so on. Your health is central to every area of your life. The state of your health will directly impact the quality of your life.

- *What value do you place on having good health, on feeling vibrant and full of vitality, and being able to perform at your peak potential?*
- *Are you listening to your body as it is communicating with you throughout each day?*
- *Do you know what your body is saying?*

We live in a high tech, high expectation society — a world of increased social and political pressures and turmoil, all placing stressful and unrealistic demands on our time, energy, relationships, health, and performance. Stress, all by itself, contributes to the onset of illness and will exacerbate existing health conditions. In addition to stress, your nutritional intake is lacking healthy substances needed to keep your body running effectively. You eat in excess, you eat to fill your belly, and you eat to calm and comfort yourself. You are not eating to nourish your body. You are living life in the fast lane, rushing and trying to keep up with the demands of the day. Your time and energy are limited so you end up eating according to what is convenient, including the convenience of preparing foods in the microwave instead of using the oven.

- *How are you to begin living with good health and vitality when most of the things you are doing are lending to the breakdown and depletion of your body's resources?*
- *How do you sustain a living body when you constantly provide it with foods void of nutritional value, basically dead substances?*

You are a living "energy being" and require sources of nourishment that contain life and energy. Your body benefits from whole food sources that naturally provide you the essentials for good health and contain enzymes and antioxidants to help you offset the daily effects of oxidative stress, better known as free radical damage. It's important you pay attention to your consumption of healthy fats and avoid harmful fats called trans-fats. Hydrogenated oils, or partially hydrogenated oils, are trans-fats, which are undesired and have long-term harmful effects on cell function. Omega fatty acids are good fats necessary for brain health and healthy cell communication.

It is essential to move your body throughout the day because it is designed to move! Movement is life-enhancing. We are fluid and energetic by nature. Staying in one position for prolonged periods makes you feel stiff and your body ache. Little or no activity lends to physical decline and debility. Technology has provided great tools and advanced options for increasing activity and mobility as well as fostering sedentary lifestyle with television remote controls and computers. A simple solution for you is to start small, to move your body even if you are sitting in a chair or standing in place. Set little goals to gradually advance yourself. For overall cardiovascular health, the American Heart

Association recommends 30 minutes of moderate intensity aerobic activity 5x/wk (150 minutes).[3]

- *Are you feeling good about your health and your lifestyle?*
- *Are you ready to make positive life-enhancing changes in your life?*
- *Are you sick and tired of feeling sick and tired?*
- *Have you been stuck in a state of overwhelm, lack of confidence, lack of ambition, lack of motivation, or lack of support?*
- *Have you been letting opportunities pass you by because you were not mentally prepared, not aware, felt inadequate, or you just didn't care?*

You are not alone in how you feel. Depending on your answers to the above questions, you can consider them valid reasons to remain where you are to minimize risk of failure, avoid getting hurt, disappointed, or embarrassed OR these could be reasons to launch you into a new season, a new way of thinking, feeling, and being. It is possible to achieve and maintain good health and naturally heal your body without excessive use of medications and invasive surgeries. Speak to your doctor about your desire for healthy lifestyle changes and surround yourself with people who will love and support you as you are making positive changes in your life. Seek to have balance in all areas of your life. With increased awareness, proper nurturing and nutrition, hydration, exercise, sleep, reducing stress and effectively managing stress, you can live with fewer incidences of disease and debilitation. You must plan and prepare to eat. Put your heart into the process of preparing and consuming your foods and beverages simply by adding love and gratitude. Make it fun and enjoyable! Whenever possible, take a nap! Restful sleep and naps help you live a healthier life.

Learn more about Sleep: National Institutes of Health (NIH)
www.nhlbi.nih.gov/health/health-topics/topics/sdd/howmuch

Here is a list of suggestions I strive to follow for my own self-care:

- Make Water your beverage of choice.
- Steam, Boil, Broil, or Bake your foods.
- Get back to basics with the use of a toaster oven, steamer, and blender.
- Use the oven or toaster oven instead of the microwave to cook and heat up your foods.
- Read the labels on the bottles and packages!
- Enzymes help you to breakdown food. You can get enzymes from raw foods such as fruits and vegetables and supplements. (Talk to your doctor about specific enzyme supplement options).
- Probiotics help support your gut health.
- Reduce your intake of sugar. Be mindful of carbohydrates converting to sugar.
- Get a basic understanding of the glycemic index and acid-alkaline balance.
- Have healthy, balanced amounts of fiber and protein in your nutrition plan.
- Eat a variety of fruits and vegetables daily. Eat Organic whenever possible.
- Become mindful of the type of fats you are ingesting. Eliminate trans-fats which are hydrogenated or partially-hydrogenated oils.
- Move your body! Movement is essential to living and thriving.
- Refresh your mind. Get outdoors whenever possible. Appreciate the beauty all around you.
- Be mindful of your breathing. It is an inspiring source that sustains you.
- Have an Attitude of Gratitude each and every day.

The list of suggestions provided may be helpful for you to improve your health. It is your responsibility to be well informed about the choices you make BEFORE making them. Please be sure to talk with your doctor about your health concerns and about any changes you would like to make to improve your health. Get your doctor's advice before making any changes to your current medical or dietary program.

YOUR BEST DEFENSE IS SELF-DEFENSE
A Healthy, Balanced Body and Strong Immune System Are Your Best Defense Against Germs and Disease!

Small and Simple Decisions You Make Everyday
ADD-UP Either Way.
It's the little things that make the biggest difference
over time.

Drug Resistant strains of bacterial infections are a challenge to our healthcare system. We are seeing younger and seemingly healthy individuals, including athletes, acquire these infections without a prior history of illness. As an example, a simple cut can turn into a full-blown infection, resulting in hospitalization, amputation, and possibly death. I have witnessed the devastating and life-altering effects these diagnoses have on the individuals and their families. There is an increased risk of infection and wounds because of limited mobility, weakened immune system, and uncontrolled diabetes. In general, the healthcare system primarily focuses on managing infections from a symptomatic perspective and tends to bypass the underlying root cause which subsequently leads to recurrent infections and additional health challenges.

The inherent value that a healthy, balanced body and immune system offer to combating life-threatening health issues, and preventing or controlling infections, is the most effective and long lasting approach to a growing epidemic. High stress and poor nutritional and behavioral habits are at the root of our problems. The problems continue to grow and crisis situations mount over time. It is up to us as educated consumers, health practitioners and educators, to pursue the knowledge, apply it in our own lives, and spread the message.

Prevention of Infections Is Our Most Effective Means of Infection Control

The most effective form of prevention occurs within our bodies. "Your greatest defense is Self-Defense!"

- *What are you doing each and every day to build your immune system?*
- *What are you doing to assist your body in offsetting the oxidative stress that occurs as a by-product of normal metabolism?*

The addition of emotional or physical stress in your life increases oxidative stress in the body. A strong immune system is your greatest asset and built-in self-defense mechanism against disease and infections. I ask for your attention to learn as much as you can, ask the necessary questions, and take action to equipping yourself and your family so that you are not taken by surprise by some unforeseen health crisis. I challenge you to make good health a way of life. In doing so, not only will you feel good, but you can offer the best of yourself to your family, friends, and community. The choice is always yours.

Learn more about Nutrition and Healthy Living:
Choosemyplate.gov
Diabetes.org
Heart.org

REFLECTION

Reflection is a vital component to effective learning and advancing one's knowledge and skill set. It is an active and purposeful process that directly ties to critical thinking. The components of reflection: reflection on action, reflection in action, and reflection for action described in the book, *Handbook of Teaching and Learning for Physical Therapists,*[4(p.192)] provides a comprehensive perspective on critical thinking and clinical reasoning. The rationale for the choices we make with regards to patient care and interactions, the amount of time we allot to prepare or recap on our experiences, the awareness we have of ourselves with respect to a given situation can be captured and examined in the reflective process. Reflection is an explorative process that can offer insight to why we make certain decisions, it is an objective method to review and assess outcomes of our decisions, and a valuable tool to plan for future decisions and actions. Without the reflective process, we close ourselves off to new learning, objectivity, personal and professional growth and development—habits develops and we continue to do things without regard to the appropriateness or subtle consequences of our actions. We unconsciously disengage and the possibility of doing things in a different way or possibly a more efficient manner is bypassed or simply dismissed.

During the time I spent working on my Doctorate in Physical Therapy, reflection became an essential part of my daily routine. It was a daily decision and still is today to persevere with optimism and enthusiasm as a way to constructively utilize my energy to effectively get through the day with a derived sense of meaning and purpose. There were unexpected challenges and significant changes in the workplace beyond my control that affected me both personally and professionally. I made every effort to consciously practice what I normally teach and strive to model in the rehab environment, the practice of mindfulness and patience in the moment as the moment arises. I found myself chuckling out loud at times because adversity seemed to be constantly rearing its head and some of it was so outrageous. It was important for me to recognize that these exact experiences I am sharing, was actually an opportunity to grow; grow deeper in my conviction and purpose for pursuing an advanced degree. It was also important for me to remember my underlying "why" which inspired my commitment. I had a desire to assist people to effectively deal with the uncertainties of life, to help them delve deeper with self-inquiry, and to acknowledge a bigger purpose for their lives. Gratitude was my saving grace along with keeping my vision of successfully completing my Doctorate in sight. A useful tool for me during this time was Motivational Interviewing (MI). I was introduced to this communication style several years ago. I was really glad to see it appear in the curriculum because I know that as we personally become aware of and practice MI, it is through the repeated eliciting and listening for "change talk" with our patients we learn to pick up on our own internal dialogue.

What I learned through this period of time that it was ok to ask for help and not allow embarrassment or shame to get in the way, to not give up or drop out because of feeling doubtful, fearful, or overwhelmed. These challenging experiences of long hours engaging in patient care, parenting, and coursework alongside the thoughtfulness and support of my teachers and classmates helped deepen my commitment and made every day and every precious moment more meaningful.

We all have felt the effects of time pressures at some point in our lives. Some of these pressures are often from our own making. We can make the effort to reduce the adverse impact of such stressors on our health by effective preparation. The preparation process starts by genuine concern and thoughtfulness for our well-being and the well-being of others. Planning ahead, allowing the opportunity for cooperation and collaboration, and creatively fostering a way to work at a steady and engaging pace may reduce some of the challenges of time pressures. How we organize and prepare in order to teach and support others have influence on outcomes. The perspective we have on the quality of our time, energy, thought, and heart that goes into preparing for the success we seek for our students, patients, clients, employees and for ourselves matters. This awareness is invaluable.

I discovered a new found appreciation for inquiry and curiosity through reflection. I was reminded through my course work how important questions are to the teaching and learning process. The quality of the questions we ask ourselves as well as the questions we ask of others really matter. The term Meta-Cognition came up in our required reading which was a relevant and useful concept that helped to validate my reasoning and efforts for the decision I had made to go back to school. The meta-cognitive process helps us to be more mindful as it is a practice and involves self-inquiry yet is often not considered until there is a problem. The process allows us to examine the breadth and depth of our thinking. It is an opportunity to explore our behaviors, feelings, and thoughts; reflect to gain insight and expand knowledge and possibly experience a deeper level of engagement in life.

The following is a relevant quote worth sharing, especially when it comes to teaching:

"Each time I walk into a classroom, I can choose the place within myself from which my teaching will come, just as I can choose the place within my students toward which my teaching will be aimed. I need not teach from a fearful place: I can teach from curiosity or hope or empathy or honesty, places that are as real within me as are my fears. I can have fear, but I need not be fear—if I am willing to stand someplace else in my inner landscape."

~Parker Palmer

Leadership is important in healthcare. Self-leadership is about personal responsibility, taking ownership for our daily decisions and experiences in life, and recognizing the potential impact we can have on the lives around us. We are interacting with people every day that can help us to examine the core of who we are and the reasoning behind what we do. People are influential "resources" that can directly or indirectly help shape and expand our thinking... help to integrate our minds and hearts, develop and reflect on our clinical thinking and reasoning skills, and put meta-cognitive knowledge into clinical practice. When all is said and done, all around us are reservoirs of information, resources we can access when needed. There is always opportunity to learn new concepts, gain insight, learn more about ourselves, and develop confidence in our ability to be a leader. We can be mentors and role models for each other through examples of personal leadership.

See Yourself In The Reflection: An Overview of Life

The influences of our environment lend to the conscious and subconscious programming of our lives, including the time developing in our mother's womb. This sets the stage for the development of our belief systems and perceptions, which serve as the foundation of our truth as we perceive it. Our subsequent choices and decisions stem from this base of perceived rationality and reality.

The fear, pain, and disappointment of the past can hold us hostage or paralyze our thoughts and actions, significantly impacting our day-to-day lives and we don't even know it. Many of us consciously or unconsciously choose to hold on to the past. We tend to hold on or numb ourselves to it until we can sense true validation of the depths of our suffering—validation of the depths of our pain, the fact that we didn't deserve it. There can be guilt that heavily weighs on our hearts as we deny our own self-forgiveness, as well as the desperate need to really let go and forgive others who have violated the very core of our being.

Counseling and talking about our problems can be helpful for a reasonable period of time but we must realize that way too much time is spent analyzing and reliving the past, wanting and seeking answers to questions that may not necessarily have a definitive answer. In this process of analysis, much of our time and energy is spent dwelling and seeking to find ourselves and to validate our sense of worth, while at the same time feeling a need for retribution for having been wronged. We get so caught up that we miss out on living right now, not recognizing that we have the opportunity to create a future that we desire and deserve—starting from our actions right where we are today.

There is a reason why people do what they do. It is usually repetition of behaviors that are learned and familiar, even if the behavior is hurtful and destructive to oneself or others. The bully and the victim are familiar examples. This cycle of behavior, commonly used as a way to build ourselves up and establish control, is actually rooted in fear and insecurity, and is tearing and wearing us down. Because of an unstable foundation, there is a great deal of spiritual, emotional, mental, and physical pain that has led to anguish and turmoil in this world. We continue to pass on the same poor examples from generation to generation. We witness the manifestation of dependencies, addictions, abusive and extreme behaviors, intolerances, self-esteem and identity issues, and in-depth psychosocial issues as a result of this generational hand-me-down. The vicious cycle of pain and dysfunction will continue until we become aware of our behavior and decide to stop it once and for all.

Perceptions of "self" have been ingrained from our early beginnings, from our circle of influences — the environment in which our young and impressionable self learns to love through examples of love. This period of development is critical and fundamental for the nurturing, shaping, and influencing of our perception of self — our perception as we relate to our environment and our world. We either develop a healthy self-identity, and learn how to trust ourselves and others through experiences of love and compassion, or we develop an insecure self-identity, and lack the ability to trust because of early experiences of pain and suffering. These early learned perceptions become the lens through which we view our life and all our relationships. Once we are aware of this profound realization, we recognize the powerful impact and life-changing effect our perspective has on every aspect of our life.

- *What really matters to you?*
- *How do you view life?*
- *What are your practices, attitudes, beliefs, feelings, and behaviors?*
- *Do you self-monitor and objectively observe your life?*

The quality of your relationships and the quality of your health matters…

- *Do you find yourself struggling in life?*
- *Do you have health or relationship challenges that require frequent doctor visits, surgeries, medications, or long-term psychology sessions?*
- *Have you engaged in or been subject to substance, emotional, or physical abuse?*
- *Do you find yourself behaving in extremes, extremes in thoughts or actions whether excessive and compulsive or repressive, regressive, and oppressive behaviors?*
- *Do your actions have you engaging in a "no tolerance" approach, an "avoidance" approach, or a "door mat" approach?*

I believe that we are here in this world to learn how to connect with one another through the experiences and purity of unconditional love—to know what it is to give and receive love in abundance. Instead, what we see and experience is a world yearning and starving for the bare essentials of unconditional love, attention, and acceptance. Love is a nurturing and invigorating resource, critical to the healthy development of our sense of self-worth. A foundation of unconditional love enables us to trust, show compassion and empathy, and helps us to engage in healthy, thoughtful relationships. We are able to sense safety and peace; we can rest and root our hearts and souls—deeply connecting to an empowering source of love and purpose.

The child that lives in all of us wants a little validation, to know that we are loved and worthy "just because." We, as individuals, as families, as a community, and as a nation, are so desperately in need of healing. We have within us a loving, powerful, Divine source for healing that is ever-present and ever-lasting. We have a way to tap into the reality of our own personal truths—innate truths that allow us to begin healing our lives and our souls. Because of the interconnectedness of all living beings, including plants and animals, our individual healing can collectively reso- nate and radiate outward to assist others in healing their wounds and discovering their own inherent truths and values. Your pres- ence and purpose is greater than what you could ever imagine.

"Being unwanted, unloved, uncared for, for- gotten by everybody, I think that is a much greater hunger, a much greater poverty than the person who has nothing to eat."

~ Mother Teresa

CALL TO ACTION

I am calling individuals, communities, businesses, and our nation to Act On Your Health. I am referring to TOTAL HEALTH… The physical, emotional, mental, and spiritual body—Health for the individual and their families, health in the work place, health in schools, health in the community, and the collective health of our nation. There is need for greater consciousness and conscien- tiousness in our day to day interactions. It's imperative that we commit to living pro-actively with continuous improvement in personal and professional knowledge and awareness. Prevention is key! It's time to recognize and pay closer attention to the influences that shape our beliefs and perceptions, which ultimately affect our choices and decisions. Let us open our hearts and minds to new ideas and concepts. We can develop healthier perceptions and insights to foster change, personal growth, and personal development. Let us take full responsibility for our lives through self-leadership. Let us develop leaders and mentors all around us through positive, inspired examples of excellence in service. Living by the Golden Rule can lend to the sincerity of human connection, the achievement of desired outcomes, and improve the overall quality of our lives.

- *Are you eager and ready to make positive, lasting change in your life?*
- *What really matters to you, your family, or your organization?*

Let us get to the root of what really matters. As parents, practitioners, educators, executives, and role models, we must first be the model of change and the positive example we want to see in others.

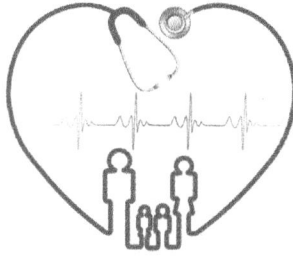

CHAPTER 2

LEADING HEALTH INDICATORS

DETERMINANTS OF HEALTH ACROSS LIFE STAGES

The public health challenge to identify what makes some people healthy and others unhealthy is a combination of subjective and objective components along with the perspectives unique to the individual and the collective perspectives of all persons involved.

- *The over arching question and desire is how can we create a nation of people where everyone has an opportunity to live a long and healthy life?*

Healthy People 2020[1] is a large set of health initiatives and objectives created to address the relationship between health status and biology, individual behavior, health services, social factors, and policies. The framework for *Healthy People 2020* was developed through an extensive collaborative process under the leadership of the Federal Interagency Workgroup (FIW).

Healthy People 2020 includes 42 focus areas with more than 1200 objectives.[2] It provides a comprehensive set of 10-year national goals and objectives that address both individual and population-level determinants of health and respective interventions towards disease prevention and health promotion. We continue to have many public health challenges, however, over the last decade there has been reported improvement in life expectancy at birth and decreased rates of death from coronary heart disease and stroke.

Many of the *Healthy People 2020* objectives focus on designing interventions that can reduce or eliminate illness, disability, and premature death. Broader focus areas include the elimination of health disparities, improving access to quality health care, strengthening public health services, addressing social determinants of health, and improving the availability and dissemination of health-related information.

In efforts to better track progress, from *Healthy People 2020* initiatives, a subset of 26 objectives was identified as high-priority health issues. This focused set of objectives was termed, *Healthy People 2020* Leading Health Indicators (LHIs).[3] These indicators are in place to help improve national health assessment, facilitate collaborative efforts, and motivate action on community, state, and national levels to improve our nation's health.

Many public health challenges still exist along with significant health disparities. The interrelationships of biological, social, economic, and environmental factors have a huge influence on individuals and communities working to make progress with selected health indicators.[4] It is essential to identify and address these major factors or determinants in order to highlight strategic opportunities to help eliminate health disparities and improve health and quality of life at any stage along the continuum.

The LHIs recognizes health from a perspective across life stages; that specific risk factors for disease and determinants for health will vary throughout the lifespan and with time. Cultivating individual and public awareness and self-care can prove to be viable strategies for early intervention and also appropriate interventions at specific points along the life course to help prevent or reduce risk of injury, illness, and disease and promote health.

Overarching Goals Healthy People 2020[1]:
- Attain high-quality, longer lives free of preventable disease, disability, injury, and premature death.
- Achieve health equity, eliminate disparities, and improve the health of all groups.
- Create social and physical environments that promote good health for all.
- Promote quality of life, healthy development, and healthy behaviors across all life stages.

DEFINING HIGH QUALITY HEALTH CARE

Quality improvement efforts in health care include targeting structure, processes, and outcome measures. The biggest area of focus regarding efforts for quality improvement is on process measures for assessment of specific patient-clinical interactions and transactions that can improve outcomes.[5] Outcome measures are endpoint measures which take into account quality of life, morbidity and mortality. This measure involves the highest complexity and is of greatest interest to clinicians and patients. There are many variances in outcomes that may not be readily modifiable and considered attributable to patient and environmental factors.

From my experiences in health care, reimbursement and evidenced based studies base their decisions and actions from outcomes. Working in various roles in a multitude of patient care environments provided me access to different touch points which have given me greater appreciation and insight for the overview of processes which lead to outcomes. To further this discussion, direct contact or interaction from a provider, practitioner, facility, or payer that involves the patient's care is referred to as a "touch point" and has specific duties and responsibilities as part of the process which leads to a specific designed goal/outcome. This process is simply a part of the whole, which I have observed has been willing to compromise the whole in order to achieve their outcomes.

The overarching vision of care is a continuum of care that involves multiple "snap shots" in time, "touch" points, and outcomes. Transition along this continuum requires seamless, accurate, and comprehensive interdisciplinary communication and collaboration at every touch point. From personal and professional experiences, observations, and conversations the original big vision of care gets lost during the transition from touch point to touch point due to multiple individualized agendas and expectations. This is a huge challenge for achieving high quality care. The "care" process has become a diluted, deceptive, and compromised system for individual gain with each entity being self-serving. Communication is ineffective and frequently incomplete or inaccurate. There are gaps at all these points in time which compromise care due to misinformation, omission, or dilution which affect the quality of care and the big vision outcome.

Heart-focused leadership efforts are needed to refresh and reform our system. Let us redefine, create new measures, implement innovative strategies and practices and accurately report in support of truly fostering high quality of care.

HEALTHCARE INNOVATION

I read an interesting article on the subject of healthcare innovation which supports a perspective I have on this matter. In efforts to shift to patient-centered and value-based services, healthcare innovation that focuses on the care model and considers processes will take the lead in guiding our focus and attention. Information technology will be the common thread for both these innovations. It is my belief that setting up for the win-win will require improving interdisciplinary flow of communication, connection through interaction and engagement, considerations for time constraints and pressures. Innovation is not simply about improving on current practices, it is the willingness to step outside of familiarity to think outside the box as we forge a new way forward. Innovation is sparked by passion and purpose to deliberately create change, to create a new process or model with greater efficiency and effectiveness typically in times when something is not working or has not yet been created.

A reference to the concept of "Design Thinking" found in the article "Defining Healthcare Innovation," by Berkowitz,[6] stated that it involved three main phases. These phases are discovery, incubation, and acceleration. In the discovery phase, the problem is studied, observed and then brainstorming occurs for solutions. In the incubation phase, there is rapid prototyping and piloting to quickly and inexpensively discover what fails and what works. For the acceleration phase, the identified successful pilot is then dispersed using a variety of techniques. Passion, time and resources are essential components to support health innovation. In addition, successful innovation requires a sustainable business model. It should integrate and support greater efficiency and effectiveness with communication and clinical workflows, and information technologies for an ever evolving healthcare system.

ENVISION THESE QUALITIES FOR YOUR ORGANIZATION

PROGRAM:
INTEGRITY • INNOVATIVE • RELIABLE • PROFITABLE
MEASURABLE • SUSTAINABLE • RESILIENT

PROCESS:
SIMPLE • PRACTICAL • REPEATABLE • CLINICAL
RELEVANCE • COLLABORATIVE • ENGAGING •
EMPATHIC • REWARDING • INSPIRING

Leading by example is one great way for practitioners to promote healthy behaviors and positive life-style changes, however, engaging and motivating our nation to making better choices involves new and effective ways of connecting and communicating with patients and the public. It requires that we have time, patience, empathy, and energy to understand the challenges and learn what interests and motivates them. It requires engaging them and guiding them to take personal responsibility to create the health and life they want. Including outside sources such as health coaches, exercise specialists, nutritionists, behavioral specialists, psychologists, or health clubs can be very helpful to support the practitioner and patient by creating a community of support and accountability partnerships.

The current practices in health care are to treat or manage diseases, however, it is not sufficient to merely manage diseases and their symptoms without also stepping back to identify the root causes and put attention on preventative measures. There are opportunities throughout the continuum of medical care where physicians and other health providers can intervene on behalf of the present and future health of their patients by providing preventative health education on healthy lifestyle options and offer supportive resources to help sustain daily efforts. A study published in the *Clinical Journal of Sports Medicine*[7] identified that the likelihood of physicians counseling on physical activity and healthier life-enhancing behaviors was influenced by the physician's own personal practice. In general, the lack of time, knowledge and experience were identified as barriers to these health promoting discussions during the course of medical care. Identifying innovative and collaborative ways to increase physician counseling on physical activity[8] during regular visits is an important objective to shifting to a preventative model of care and restoring effectiveness in quality of care and health outcomes.

Time demands and constraints affect us in every area of our lives and businesses. Truthfully, as it relates to health care delivery, it only takes a few seconds for a physician to write the prescription. The real time challenge is in educating the patient on the true value of exercise, identifying motivations and barriers, and then following-up. If you as the practitioner are not personally motivated to engage in healthy activities and do not have the support staff in place, this would not be a likely priority.

An example of innovative thinking is from a Model Physician Leader who started a local activity called "Walk with a Doc"[9] which has now gained popularity and become a national movement. Another great example of an innovative resource is the site Exercise Is Medicine®[10] which was co-launched in 2007 by the American Medical Association (AMA) and the American College of Sports Medicine (ACSM). It is has since expanded to a global initiative managed by the ACSM. This site provides education on incorporating regular physical activity (PA) into your lifestyles and supports doctors in prescribing exercise for their patients. The initiative for Physical Activity and exercise as a vital sign is gaining support.[11,12]

HEALTHCARE CHALLENGES AND CONCERNS

An enormous amount of time, energy, money, and resources have been invested into improving our healthcare system in the United States. There are still many questions to the direction in which public and private sectors are heading. The slow pace of improving quality care and reducing health care costs raises concerns for the future. It is imperative that we reexamine our policies, procedures, and processes from a collaborative approach, one that is truly interdisciplinary. We are striving to do more with less and this model of care is NOT working. As a health professional working in this system for over two decades, I can share that my challenges today are greater to keep up with the unrealistic and sometimes ridiculous expectations that interfere with the intended purpose for delivering quality, safe, and effective care.

I feel it is absolutely critical we look at the political and procedural choices being made in healthcare. I have come to recognize there are "rotten apples" in this system on every level which presents us with ethical concerns and the need to prevent and account for fraud, misuse, and abuse. I believe that basic operational requirements to deliver honest, cost effective, and quality care has to start with looking at how we define and support care from all touch points in this system. "We" as system stakeholders require a shared vision and set of principles and practices that include innovative strategies and actions for improving communication processes and facilitating "flow" in the delivery and documentation of care, and include efficient and effective technological solutions that are engaging, sensitive and supportive to the needs of patients, providers, payers, and investors.

Considerations for health literacy are critical to the quality and effectiveness of health care delivery. Low health literacy is a challenge to health care outcomes as it impacts effective communication, health promotion, proper self-care and medical management. The United States has more than 1 in 3 adults with low health literacy.[13] This finding lends support to the potential adverse affects low health literacy has on the quality and cost of health care and possible barrier to the overall quality of care.

For individuals with low health literacy, there is less understanding of health conditions and there is greater chance for medication errors. Collaborative efforts to identify individual needs for communication and comprehension are an essential component to the initial health assessment. Due to typical time constraints, use of a quick screening test can help to assess health literacy.[13] Communication can be delivered with pictures, single word or few simple words at a time, or by having the patient show you or repeat back to you for clarification what they heard and understand. Involve family when available to support this process. Cultural considerations are important for an accurate health literacy assessment. Be sensitive, as it is important to not stigmatize or embarrass anyone in this process.

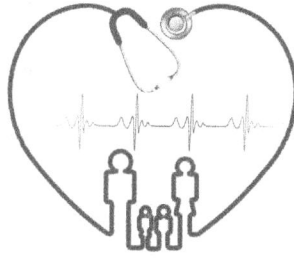

CHAPTER 3

THE ROAD AHEAD

HEALTHCARE PRIORITIES AND RECOMMENDATIONS

It is time to make good health a priority with new resolve to take responsibility and practice healthier habits. This is an invitation for a new pace of living well, for an immediate shift from the current broken, disease and disability focus to a health promoting, self-awareness, and self-empowerment focus through education on the benefits of self-care practices and self-management training that educates and empowers adults and adolescents to develop the knowledge, skills, and motivation to make healthier life-enhancing choices, improve health behaviors, and increase a sense of overall well-being. Physicians and other health professionals are uniquely positioned to regularly provide patient education and encouragement on exercise, proper nutrition, and other lifestyle interventions that are key players in the prevention, treatment, and management of chronic disease.

The World Health Organization (WHO) predicts that by the year 2020, seven out of 10 deaths will be attributed to non-communicable diseases such as heart disease, diabetes, cancer and respiratory disease and that these diseases are preventable with effective strategies and actions to deal with their associated risk factors.[1] It is essential that we develop relationships and alliances through collaborative efforts with organizations, schools, businesses, and community leaders to create awareness and identify supportive resources for the delivery of relevant and cost-effective and cost-saving self-care management trainings.

Engaging in healthy behaviors has been scientifically supported as a way to prevent and treat chronic diseases, however, public health concern and the financial burden continues to rise as there are millions of people living with obesity and associated non-communicable chronic diseases. Chronic disease practice guidelines call for lifestyle change as the first course of treatment, however, it is identified that less than half of primary care physicians in the United States routinely provide specific guidance on physical activity, nutrition, or weight management.[2] One main reason for this is the lack of formal educational and health promotion counseling in medical school. Inclusion of lifestyle medicine (LM) curriculum in medical education is a critical and strategic move that can assist in getting to the root cause of many of our chronic disease challenges and health care costs.[2,3] The integration of LM competencies throughout medical education is expected to have important public health implications. This type of training offers a scalable and sustainable model to educate physicians using evidenced based curriculum on how to effectively guide and promote healthy lifestyle choices for the prevention and treatment of lifestyle related diseases.[2,3] This training will hopefully also engage medical students in their own self-care and behavior change to sustain good health and by personal example support their patients to do the same.

Self-Management Support Can Improve Patient Outcomes and Control Costs

- *Are you taking care of yourself as you care for others?*
- *Is living healthy a priority in your life?*
- *Do you realize that your health affects EVERY aspect of your life and the lives of those around you?*

Most illnesses and deaths attributed to chronic diseases are preventable. At state and national levels, public health concerns and challenges are of great priority. There are numerous behavioral factors associated with the development of chronic illness. The intention is that with the efforts on education and reducing health disparities, much of the chronic disease burden may be reduced. A positive change in self-care behavior is necessary for preventing future health problems and can also help with effectively managing long-term conditions. Daily self-care behaviors and lifestyle habits are critical elements for preventative health care as well as disease management. It is important to consider how one copes with illness and deals with stress and emotions that affect overall health and well-being. Deliberate and strategic self-care practices and interventions can have significant impact on health and health care costs over the course of time.

Dealing with human behavior, beliefs, and attitudes is a challenge. Habits and patterns of behavior start very early in life and lead to lifestyle choices that affect one's health for a lifetime. From experiences in the acute rehab setting, the desire or motivation for change often happens after a significant life-altering event. Individuals can learn to live well through the implementation of self-care management tips and strategies. There are programs and hopefully with the support of this book that will provide useful and practical information to empower and motivate towards healthier lifestyle choices leading to a happier and healthier way of life.

An interesting study on the long-term effects of a 3-day residential body awareness program (BAP) conducted at the Lifestyle Training Center in the Netherlands identified that the participants were better able to cope with stress, had positive behavior changes, and had improved ability to manage their health problems up to twelve months after the program ended without additional intervention.[4] During this period of time participants developed increased body awareness, increased self-efficacy, were better able to express emotions, had a less depressive style, had a reduction in psychosomatic symptoms, and reported an increase in quality of life.

This study[4] provides evidence to support the extended benefits of a short term self-management training that focuses attention on body awareness and building self-efficacy. With this type of intervention, patient educators may be able to increase their effectiveness with helping patients manage psychosomatic symptoms associated with chronic health problems. Employers, health insurance companies, and society benefit from early intervention of successfully implemented short-term, cost-effective programs. Programs such as this provide viable options for physician referral.

HEALTH LITERACY AND ADHERENCE

It has been part of my ongoing education to better understand the need for rehabilitation professionals to consider the health literacy of their patients as it directly relates to compliance / adherence and outcomes. This topic was mentioned in a health promotion review I performed for the state of Nevada. It mentioned the increased risk for chronic disease based on low level of education or literacy. As healthcare providers, we are in key positions to influence positive lifestyle changes and long-term outcomes for our patients through our genuine concern, knowledge, and the quality of time spent during patient care interactions. Screening or assessment of how to best educate and support our patients is typically through the rapport we build, the specific questions we ask, as we look at patients from a perspective of their overall well-being. Asking general questions that draw on their interests, lifestyles, and motivations should be part of the subject interview as well as how they learn best.

Education is an important component throughout any hospital stay. Admissions education can help orient new patients and their families to a facility. In the acute rehab environment, this early education is included as part of therapy. I love this period of time because I have an opportunity to help engage patients in their rehabilitation process. At this point in time I can help lay the ground work for opening lines of communication, establish what the patient's perspectives are around the immediate care and goals for rehab, and discuss the personal responsibility that comes as part of whatever the expressed goals may be for the short period of time in the rehabilitation facility. I can honestly report that when we ask questions about perspective, the response tends to elicit a broad range of perspectives based on each patient's experience prior to rehab. This includes fears and concerns, and whether patients have an understanding of why they are in rehab and if they have support at this time in their life. There is a great deal of change that takes place after a life-altering accident or illness that can shake a person up and also wake them up to doing better and doing differently.

As healthcare providers and clinicians, it is our responsibility to provide patients, families, and caregivers with accurate and understandable information to help them effectively manage their condition. Information can be disease specific, or specific to pain management on the use of medications or other methods of pain control and how to effectively communicate with clinicians about pain responses and the medications they receive for pain management. It is essential that we encourage autonomy by giving our patients the opportunity to express what works best for them during any given day. As providers, it is our responsibility to look, listen, feel, and ask questions of all of our patients and get to know our patients. Knowing where they have been, as far as their experiences, and where they want to go is very helpful in identifying what motivates or distracts them from maximizing their functional gains. A skillful and thoughtful assessment of the patient's functionality includes cognition, safety awareness, awareness of his/her health condition and precautions, discussion around perspectives on hospitalization/rehab, identifying needs, likes, dislikes, and personal and salient goals. It is important to establish and discuss a game plan and reinforce a team effort with the patient being the main player in the process.

There are various options for how we identify patient preference for learning, language needs, and cultural variances. There are handouts, verbal instruction, and interpreters by phone or in person to assist with patient education. We can also utilize family support and education as part of the education process and follow-up.

A Closer Look At Health Literacy

Attention to health literacy is a major concern in health care as it directly affects how we deal with public health challenges. Research by Kripalani et al[5] on "Health Literacy and the Quality of Physician-Patient Communication During Hospitalization," defined health literacy as the ability for the individual to obtain, process, understand, and act on basic health information and services needed to make appropriate health decisions. They indicated that low health literacy was linked to low self-efficacy. For this population, they also identified there was less physician interaction with the patient and frequent use of medical terms the patient was not able to understand that could contribute to poor physician-patient communication. It is important to consider that patients may have challenges learning about their condition because of difficulty reading or understanding written information, including difficulty reading prescription drug labels. There may also be a lack of confidence when patients have to fill out forms by themselves.

In general, what I have noticed in healthcare is that we give a lot of information in a short period of time, especially at time of discharge. This is an automatic set-up for miscommunication, poor understanding, and non-compliance especially with medication management. This is something I feel needs to be addressed in the way of our processes that can definitely be improved upon. It is a difficult enough process for patients to work on healing when in the hospital as they are simultaneously trying to absorb all the information coming in from various sources. The stress that accompanies the situation confounds the ability to fully process and comprehend information.

- *Even with average or above average health literacy, when you are feeling sick or bothered by something, how attentive or focused are you?*

Frustration, overwhelm, and confusion are a few typical factors that coincide with healthcare whether it is a simple visit to the doctor or a life-altering situation in the hospital. The complications and considerations for people with low health literacy get more complex due to these normal factors as part of the human experience. It is important for us to keep in mind that low health literacy touches on personal and cultural sensitivity, and supportive efforts to reduce stigma and embarrassment can foster open lines of communications and appreciation.

Research reports that 40% of adults in the United States are dealing with low health literacy and that people with low health literacy have higher incidence of hospitalization and higher mortality rates.[5] They identified that the quality of communication between the physician and patient had affects on outcomes; that poor physician-patient communication can affect readmission rates and may contribute to adverse events after discharge. In the study,[5] eight domains were used in a post-discharge questionnaire:

1. General clarity
2. Responsiveness to patient concerns
3. Explanation of patients' problems
4. Explanation of processes of care
5. Explanation of self-care after discharge
6. Empowerment
7. Decision making
8. Consideration of patients' desire and ability to comply with recommendations.

This particular study had 84 patients who each completed an in-hospital interview and phone interview after discharge. Forty-four percent of patients in this study were identified as having inadequate health literacy. Results showed that the overall poorest ratings for physician communication were in consideration of patients' desire and ability to comply with recommendations. Significantly worse ratings by patients with inadequate health literacy were in the domains of general clarity, responsiveness to patient concerns, and explanation of processes of care.

People with limited health literacy have greater difficulty with following medical instructions, are more likely to misunderstand health information, have greater physical and mental health issues, have higher rates of hospitalization and shorter life expectancy.[6] As a practitioner, I recognize the importance of effective communication being a huge component to how we deliver care, the patient's perceived value of care, and the overall quality of care.

The bottom line is that the patient experience matters and considerations for health literacy will impact this experience as well as quality of care and quality of life outcomes. Patients need time to express their concerns and deserve clear explanations about their medical care. If a patient's literacy skills are identified as being limited, extra time and care, and special considerations may be needed to support communication. Efforts to effectively manage the challenges of health literacy may include the use of simple, plain language with education materials and patient consent forms, use of visual aids, use of a communication method referred to as "teach back" to identify patient understanding, and provide health professional education on health literacy.[6]

Two specific studies[7,8] on screening for limited health literacy in the *Journal of General Internal Medicine* have validated ONE specific screening question as being useful in detecting patients with inadequate healthy literacy.

"How confident are you filling out medical forms by yourself?"

It is important to consider the response answers to the questions asked of patients to ensure complete understanding. Wording of the answers in the VA study[8] were slightly modified to help improve the participant's understanding of the questions: "Instead of *always, often, sometimes, occasionally,* or *never,* participants were asked to choose between all of the time, most of the time, some of the time, a little of the time or none of the time."

PERSON-CENTERED HEALTH CARE
Advocacy in Health Care Delivery

It is easy to see how communication can break down inviting problems and misunderstandings, or how upset and dissatisfaction can arise when health care seems impersonal, when you as the patient do not feel seen or heard. The focus on disease management instead of patient-focused care occurs far more often than it should. My first-hand experiences as a health professional and having loved ones in a hospital has prompted my interest and position as a healthcare advocate for human issues and healthcare processes.

Knowledge of health and disease is a necessity for competent delivery of care, however, the ability to openly and empathically listen, ask open ended questions to elicit patient response and understanding, be genuine in your concern for the well-being of the person, engage the patient in his/her own process, and have the sensitivity to tune into non-verbal aspects of communication are just as important if not more so for the long term impact of the experience.

Patient-centered care encourages shared control between the patient and practitioner in decision-making about interventions or management of the illness or situation. The consultation or interaction focuses on the patient as a whole person, not merely a disease or body part.[9] The patient's perspective of the provider's sincere attentiveness and concern helps to cultivate a positive experience which ultimately creates the kind healing environment that supports the desired goals and outcomes.

Problems with communication can arise when healthcare providers focus on the disease rather than caring for the person.[9] Patient-centered behavior is a skill that can be developed that affects patient satisfaction and may likely influence health outcomes. Training interventions that have condition-specific materials for health provider training and patient education may have beneficial effects on health behavior and health status.[9] I believe that as an adjunct to any training intended for healthcare providers is to simultaneously cultivate a mindset of advocacy. This patient-centered approach can prove to be relatively simple, collaborative, broad spread, effective, and rewarding if all healthcare providers were to view themselves as patient advocates in their daily work.

COLLABORATIVE CARE IS MEDICINE
The Therapeutic Alliance:
Being Fully Present

Genuinely Caring

Empathic Listening

> Establish Rapport
>
> Build Trust
>
> Alleviate Fears and Concerns
>
> Promote Autonomy
>
> Shared Goals and Vision

Collaborative care is much a part of the healing process therefore can be included in the prescription for health. Collaborative care begins with the practitioner–patient relationship and building trust. This collaboration has a minimum of two people acknowledging the same desired goals with a network of support and resources to help attain and sustain those goals. The relationship matters. It is about us working together, aligning efforts for common purposes, goals, and outcomes. It is an exchange that can have involved parties feeling empowered and enriched versus feeling disabled and helpless. It is a symbiotic relationship which ties into a network of symbiotic relationships rallying around the same purpose and goal. It is the perspective that, "What matters to you matters to me." Whether we are the patient, practitioner, or caregiver we all want to be seen, heard and validated. It is essential that we remove the demand mentality of fix me or listen to me, do what I say or else... True collaborative medicine fosters the kind of dialogue amongst all persons interacting to care for a patient that allows us to see and appreciate the "whole person" not just a patient with a certain diagnosis or the patient in the bed or the body part on the operating table.

The delivery process includes the information itself along with the "deliverer" of information. From my professional observation and practice, it is essential and more effective when health education is perceived by the patient as being relevant, helps engage the patient in his/her own healthcare process, and is communicated at a pace and literacy level that the patient will be better able to grasp and understand. We are facilitators, coaches and mentors, the patient's guide at the side. Collaborative efforts will begin with reaching internally to genuinely care about the desired outcome in order to gain the patient's trust and gather insights to individual motivations for personal goals and desires for successful outcomes. In addition, collaborative efforts are supported and reinforced by interdisciplinary efforts in facilities, in homes by caregivers, and extend to partnerships in our local communities and abroad which expand support and resources.

Across the continuum in healthcare, we can encourage and promote physical activity as a standard baseline measure to achieving healthier outcomes. Integrating and implementing exercise in our daily life can be an effective way to prevent, treat, and manage many chronic health illnesses. The organization Exercise is Medicine® is encouraging healthcare providers to take their pledge, to assess and record physical activity (PA) as a vital sign during patient visits and then end the visit with a prescription for exercise or referral to a health professional or certified health fitness professional for follow-up counseling and support.[10]

THE OLYMPIC EDGE

While watching this year's Olympic events with great excitement and feeling honored to live in the United States, a pattern emerged for me that highlighted missing components to creating an integrative and collaborative framework we so desperately need in healthcare. I recognized that when a TEAM is dedicated and courageous as these exceptional athletes, commits and collaborates towards a clear vision with enthusiasm, passion, and disciplined practice, this organically cultivates an engaged, inspired and self-sustainable model that can exponentially exceed in performance, surpassing possibilities beyond limits to the imagination. This is testament to the familiar saying that when the team works the dream works. The Olympic Edge proposes a Collaborative-Competitive hybrid model, where competitive refers to the challenge to be great, to strive and rise to the best of our abilities, which through personal inner work and self-disciplined practices, lends individual performance contributing to the collective "whole" which accounts for the individual, the team members, and the supportive players and environment in which we are playing.

- *Can we set up for win-win outcomes?*

I believe that when we remove the titles and labels, allowing the intention for the Spirit of gratitude, honor, and humility to safely and openly meet with ego and pride the dialogue and process begins. This initiates a symbiotic type of connection through a natural internal-external process that is concurrently happening for the individual and the various participants involved in this gathering. There is an inherent sensitivity and vulnerability as we navigate through such authentic conversations, however through this "mind" field a positive and healthy relationship can emerge and we can learn to appreciate and align with our deepest core values and simultaneously cultivate a sense of cohesiveness, connectedness, conscientiousness, and contribution that first moves in us and then through us in service to a shared vision and purpose. It is in this space we get to unite the best of ourselves in thought, actions, beliefs, attitudes, and perspectives creating the desire for a win-win outcome. The team focus and interactions are all for one and one for all, we are in this together.

MINDFULNESS ON THE MOVE

- *Are you aware of the moment to moment happenings in your body?*
- *Are you listening or tuning in to the what is being communicated to you, how you are feeling in response to whatever is taking place in the moment whether externally or internally?*

Clinical Implications for Short-Term Mindfulness Meditation in Healthcare

Fostering the future success of mindfulness meditation as a "preventive and adjunctive medicine" would first encourage that doctors and practitioners support this intervention by their own personal practice.[11] Stress is one of the biggest challenges affecting medical professionals so even a brief period of mindfulness meditation can serve as an effective strategy to support self-control when our inner resources are low or depleted.[11,12] This implementation could help create a shift in perspective of how to effectively model and deliver care by the beneficial outcomes of our own practice. Doctors and health practitioners who choose to practice mindfulness meditation could better help their patients cultivate mindful behaviors as a way to improve health and well-being.

The well known 8-week Mindfulness Based Stress Reduction[13] (MBSR) model has numerous documented health benefits associated with this practice, however, the expense and lengthier time-frame are not practical and accommodating for typical healthcare environments. Shorter variations of a few days participating in mindfulness meditation can have broad range of health benefits for our patients, and is more cost-effective and versatile.[14-16] A short-term intervention of mindfulness meditation can improve mood states, reduce anxiety and fatigue and potentially enhance how we process information.[14,16] The positive findings in these studies mentioned have been in part due to the participants reported interest or motivation to participate and their expectations of the outcome.[13,17-19] An immediate effect that I have personally experienced and a commonly reported experience from my patients have been the calming effects of the practice.

Mindfulness meditation offers a unique opportunity in healthcare to serve as an adjunctive intervention in the area of mind-body medicine, functioning both as an integrative and participatory medical model of care.[19] It is a practice that cultivates present moment awareness while promoting a balance between a calm yet alert state of mind...there is focused attention and noticing of breath, thoughts, and body sensations while maintaining a relaxed, non-judgmental awareness of self and the environment.[13,20] Studies have shown that mindfulness meditation has positive physiological effects on the brain and immune function and positive effects on behavior and handling of negative emotions under stress, reducing cortisol and blood pressure.[16,19,20] Mindfulness meditation has effects on self-regulation... providing greater capacity for self-control and self-awareness, curbing reactive impulses or emotional triggers, and reducing the experience of pain with chronic pain patients.[15,17,20-22] This simple and practical tool offers us a resource to better regulate our emotions and effectively cope with life's demands.

Short-term mindfulness meditation training can be an adjunct to the care we currently provide and easily be included as part of our patient's plan of care and home exercise program. It is a versatile intervention that can be delivered to the individual or in group format in a variety of patient care settings. The desired outcome would be for patients to experience some beneficial effect whether immediately or during the short course of this training which may encourage an interest in continuing a mindfulness practice. This intervention could prove to be helpful in cultivating and promoting healthy lifestyle choices and help manage a growing population of patients with chronic illnesses.

As an adjunctive therapy, mindfulness meditation has influences on physical and emotional health and healing, however further studies in this area are needed to explore the potential benefits and effects on specific conditions and disorders. It is my belief from experiences and through studies reviewed that a mindfulness practice can support our well-being as practitioners and has an added benefit of cultivating our listening and empathic skills—helping us to develop a more compassionate and resilient approach in our personal lives and supports us in our respective work environments. The potential long-term success of this versatile, complementary medical intervention in healthcare would support healing, health and well-being, and affect quality of care and quality of life outcomes.

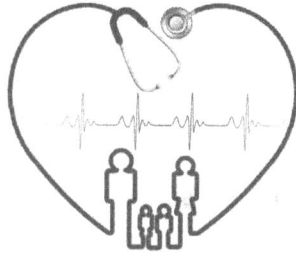

CHAPTER 4

PERSPECTIVES MATTER

HEALTH INTEGRITY

- *What is holding you together?*
- *What sustains you?*

A personal example of what I am referring to as health integrity came to me as I was lying in bed feeling very uncomfortable, back aching, and exhausted from trying to keep up with a very hectic schedule. Acknowledging that this way of feeling and being was counterproductive and counter intuitive, the word integrity came to mind. I asked myself, "What's holding me together?" The image of layers and layers of duck tape and masking tape, criss-crossed and bandaging me up somewhat like a "mummy" and continually adding more layers to hold me together, was the image that reflected in my mind but which was also being felt as a tightening around my rib cage. An inner dialogue began, "I know better, yet day after day, I am pushing myself and not supporting myself with adequate rest, nutrition and hydration…" I asked myself, "Why am I doing this and for how long will I keep this up?"

The real connection to my situation and frustration was when I sat up, my back muscles felt so tense as though I had rods running through them on either side of my spine holding me upright. I felt totally exhausted. I was running on empty and yet I was nowhere near where I wanted to be or feel. I had been struggling to get through each day…working 11-12 hours a day with the days literally running together, while only getting 2-5 hours of consecutive sleep night after night and week after week. This schedule was beginning to take a toll. I had to identify for myself, what was the real truth of my situation? I had to revisit my values and aspirations for my life.

- *Does this scenario sound familiar to you?*

When we continually push ourselves without the awareness and live life on autopilot, over time we become depleted and end up getting sick, injured, or burnt out. Common questions and statements I hear so often after a patient/family health crisis are: "How did I get here? How did this happen? What's to come of my life? Why me? I can't believe it. I didn't see it coming. I didn't realize."

Writing this book on self-care has me closely examining and reflecting on my habits, values, and daily actions and inactions. As healthcare providers and caregivers, we especially need to tune-in to our bodies as the demand is high and our resources get used up quickly. Our beliefs, perspectives, and habits play a huge role in our decisions and way of life, and our health integrity. Notice if the way you are working, the decisions you are making, and the way you are feeling aligns with what is most meaningful to you.

- *How do you spend your time, energy and resources?*
- *Are you enthusiastic about the work you do, the life you live?*
- *Are you in alignment and congruent with your core values?*
- *Are your efforts in support of your desired outcomes, the lifestyle you want, and your heartfelt desires?*

PRACTITIONER PERSPECTIVE

Implementing a great idea has it challenges. Medical complexities and vastness in perspectives present many variables to the innovation and integration process. When surveying and talking to staff, it is important to identify all who would benefit from process and cultural reforms. The inclusive criteria can be an extensive process to identify all the touch points necessary to open up conversation and better understand the patient and practitioner course of care.

Healthcare delivery is not merely about assessment and treatment using standardized protocols with an interdisciplinary approach to the plan of care, it must account for the unpredictable and sensitive nature of human interaction during this process. There are multiple processes occurring simultaneously from the organizational level to the patient level. It is important to consider the influence of each healthcare provider on patient care outcomes. This influence may include the provider's feelings, confidence, beliefs, experiences, perspectives, personal health, literacy, choice of words, knowledge, or personal bias. A realization of this for me became very apparent after starting an oncology program. The first year of the program uncovered many unanticipated variables and challenges. I recognized that an increased level of professional sensitivity, disease and treatment knowledge, and considerations for the practitioner's personal experiences and perspectives around cancer affected the rehabilitative process.

I have listened to patients and their families share their deepest heartfelt desires, express their deepest fears and uncertainties of "tomorrow." I have witnessed the angst and the sorrow when the course of rehab changed due to the decline in health sending the patient back to the hospital, palliative care, or hospice instead of home where the original intention for rehab was established as a goal. The psychosocial-emotional dynamics inherent to healthcare will challenge the provider to grow in awareness, in patience, and sensitivity. Through closely working with oncology patients, I have learned so much more about myself and have opened my heart in ways I had yet to experience. I have had the most amazing conversations and life-changing experiences with patients and their families.

To capture the fullness and depth of this type of service is challenging, as it has no clearly defined boundaries due to the vastness of perspectives and beliefs. It opens us to possibilities for the heart to experience beyond what we may have ever thought possible. Its very nature is complex, expansive, sensitive, unpredictable, and incredibly rewarding. "Sensitivity" is a heart set and a skill set, allowing us to make adjustments in the moment. As providers, as we spend time getting to know and work with patients and their families, we are simultaneously getting to know ourselves.

I am truly excited for continued growth and upward mobility with an enlightened perspective, appreciation, and greater insight and awareness to healthcare processes. It is essential to identify the gaps and gains of health care delivery at all levels. Collective awareness and dialogue around the desires and challenges of clinical operations and processes help foster an organic process...creating dynamic synergy through support networks working for successful implementation, growth, and expansion of our health care delivery system.

PATIENT PERSPECTIVE

To increase practitioner awareness and sensitivity, it is important to gather perspectives from a desirable and undesirable point of view from the patient's perspective of how care is delivered and received. There are many positive and desirable aspects to care, however, in conversations with patients over the years, I have compiled a brief list that offers some insight on the Patient's Perspective when care has been felt or perceived as undesirable:

Patient Perspectives on their Care: (Undesirable)

- Feeling emotional, embarrassed or afraid to ask or be annoying
- Don't want to bother the staff
- Personal issues being discussed in hallway
- Too much light from the hallway at night
- People are more interested in shutting off the call light than in assisting them
- CNA will say yes and not be seen again
- Noise or light at times from the bathroom
- Limited food options or do not like the food
- Limited TV channels
- Feeling roughed up first thing in the morning by the CNA with waking up and with moving to get out of bed
- Roughness in touch with cleaning up
- Tone of voice too loud and not sounding kind or caring
- Waiting an hour for help after call light is pushed
- Asked to not get out of bed without assistance—yet have to get out of bed so as not to wet or soil themselves
- Much harder to process or take in information when emotional
- Don't feel like they have a chance to ask questions
- Don't feel like they are being heard
- Don't feel like people really care, it's just their job

- People are just here for a paycheck
- It's been days, have not been able to see or talk to the doctor
- The doctor comes in when I am sleeping or half asleep for me to remember anything
- The doctor rushed in and out, I didn't have a chance to say anything
- I could not understand anything the doctor was saying

MAKE TIME TO CARE

I had an experience with a rehab patient who had motioned me to come into her room as I was walking by her door. It was obvious to me that she was upset and wanted to talk about her situation. This was the day she made a decision for hospice yet the logistics involved were perceived as too much, uncaring, and in her words not sympathetic or considerate. In her words, she cried and asked me, *"Don't they know that when a person is sick and in pain, rushing them is not helpful. Why are they doing this to me?"* She was in the midst of her own processing and preparing as we were in the midst of our processing and preparing for her discharge to another level of care.

As we know, healthcare is a business, however, the steps we take to truly care for our patients and meet the requirements of our system-imposed processes do not offer us room to flex, adjust, or offer us sufficient time without some consequence whether it is not meeting a deadline, benchmark, quota, or a personal need. I sat with her to explain the process from start to finish, where she had decisions to make earlier but was not ready to make them and the decisions we had to make based on insurance and rehab criteria were upon her now. I explained her rights, the choices she had, and addressed her questions and concerns. I also addressed her fears and disappointments that had her feeling angst about her transition. Ultimately, I provided the information and offered support to help her better understand and feel somewhat peaceful as a result of our conversation during this meaningful time together.

This type of desensitized care can be experienced by any of us. A few months ago, I received a text from my young niece while she was standing in the hospital room listening to the doctor talk to her 46 year old mother who was struggling to fight her battle with cancer. She was so upset from the face-to-face one-sided conversation the doctor was having with her mother, who was lying in the hospital bed barely responsive, repeatedly saying to his patient, "You know you aren't going to get better. You are dying." Her mom responded with moans. My niece expressed to me her anger and helplessness at this situation. The doctor proceeded to tell my niece that there was no point in trying to keep her mother alive, that medically there was nothing else to do for her, and that she needed to go to hospice. To say the least, I was furious and shocked to hear about this insensitive interaction! I could not believe these words that I was reading through this text from my niece who was clearly overwhelmed trying to process losing her mother and having to make the decision for hospice while contending with the lack of compassion and tact from the physician in charge of her mother's care.

- *If you or I were lying in that bed, how would we want this to actually play out?*
- *If this was your loved one, how would that make you feel?*
- *As a practitioner, do you recognize that your expertise over time can lead to you becoming desensitized in how you deliver the actual "care"?*

"Kindness is the language which the deaf
can hear and the blind can see."

~ Mark Twain

Man Made Misery

We create the practices, policies, processes, and politics which include expectancies, time constraints, and tolerances and we can change them. We are all customers and consumers of the health-care system.

- *Ever wonder why we feel stressed and pressured to meet the demands that we, society at large, have created?*
- *How can we create an infrastructure that considers the dynamics of a collaborative versus competitive working relationship?*
- *How do we fit sensitivity and practicality into the same process?*
- *Can we explore how to set ourselves up for a win-win solution or is there always an offensive–defensive proposition?*

"Every adversity, every failure and every
heartache carries with it the seed of an
equivalent or greater benefit."

Think and Grow Rich by Napoleon Hill[1(p.55)]

-

The quote here from Napoleon Hill can remind us that despite all the challenges we face, positive change is possible! For me, that inspires HOPE!

CONSCIENTIOUS AND COMPASSIONATE CARE
Putting the CARE Back Into Healthcare

- *Why is it we wait until end of life to provide service that ensures the maintenance of comfort, dignity, and respect?*
- *It is important that at end of life we treat people with loving, considerate care, but why isn't this happening before we are at this point; where is the same regard and concern before end of life?*

Health care has become a mechanical system, a system that has dwindled in consciousness and conscientiousness. We are missing the compassion and concern for human issues. Our health care system is overwhelmed by an increasing demand for quality care while insurance companies and medical facilities seek to reduce their expenses and maintain cost effectiveness for services they provide. There has been abuse and misuse of the system at every level and, as a result, we have a system in place that is desensitized, detached, and devaluing.

Many of us have been "buying into" a health insurance plan expecting it to assist us by covering our medical expenses and medical equipment as they arise. Most of us don't expect to need intensive acute care inpatient rehabilitative services for anything more than an elective surgical procedure.

- *What if you do require this level of care for something major and unexpected, do you qualify? How long will you be permitted to stay?*

This is an interesting process most people don't know about. There is a list of criteria to be met that allows you to qualify to receive certain services, and there is a certain level of progress and functionality, "other qualifiers," that allow you to continue receiving services. Working in an acute care rehabilitation setting, I frequently witness denials for continued service, even when a patient is making progress and despite advocating for more time. The mechanical nature of service that currently exists is doing a disservice to the well-being of our society as a whole. At every level, things need to change. *We all want to get more for less, but where is that getting us?* We have more problems, more frustration, more dissatisfaction, more disease, etc. *What does this mean for our future if we maintain this self-serving outlook?* After all, at every level, we are the customers in this system. We have to collectively change as a society; however, this has to start with the individual's outlook on personal health and personal responsibility. It is important that we step up and advocate for each other, that we do better than we are doing now; take personal interest in each other's welfare and well-being, hold each other accountable to a higher standard of living, and expect a level of personal responsibility.

Our actions and attitudes either lend to or take away from the greater whole. In order to improve our system, it's imperative we create a new philosophy and culture in our various environments—nurturing respect, appreciation, and consideration; reviving compassion and conscientiousness in our atmosphere that says we all affect one another. Let us set in motion this life supporting philosophy that will foster trust and send a message that we care. We can seek to find what is common, not fear what is different. We can unite on common ground, lessen the judgment, lesson criminal activity, and lessen suffering and victimization by extending our hands and hearts in service.

As a physical therapist, it is always important for me to recognize the vulnerability and volatility of the clients and patients who come within my sphere of influence. Whether as their evaluating therapist or treating therapist working towards their established goals, it's important for me to remember that within each person there is a personal history lurking in the background. The concerns and fears from their current illness, surgery, or incident are also accompanied by experiences, habits, and perceptions which occurred prior to their immediate situation. The process the individual will go through will vary and WE can contribute in a positive manner to this process. The awareness of one's presence is important for overall objectivity. The ability to listen, connect, empathize, and utilize our senses during patient interaction will assist in fostering trust and developing rapport.

Seek greater knowledge and appreciation of the therapeutic value of high intention, high touch...working from and through the heart to the heart.

- *What if you couldn't walk, talk, or you were paralyzed, what would that mean to you?*
- *What would it mean to not be able to move your arms and legs, not be able to move your body, not be able to eat from your mouth, instead take liquids through a feeding tube?*
- *What would a 24-hour day look and feel like if your mobility was limited and you could not care for yourself?*
- *What would it mean to you if you had to have someone help you with every aspect of your care?*
- *What if you added pain to all these mentioned conditions?*
- *How would you keep yourself from getting depressed, keep yourself from being stuck in negative or pessimistic thoughts and emotions?*
- *How can we help our patients as well as their families to overcome discouragement, despair, and disillusion?*

As practitioners, we have significant influence on our patients. I have gained a great deal of insight from my experiences working in hospitals and acute care rehabilitation facilities. I notice that many people reach a junction in life after a major surgery, major incident, or major accident. I meet them at this critical and sensitive time, a time of uncertainty and transition. I find this to be an honor and a privilege to have an opportunity to make a positive difference through a warm presence, creating a safe space for open and honest dialogue, with empathic concern and sincere interest to be of support and guidance towards achieving their personal desires and goals.

- *What happens to you and how do you feel when you, as the patient, encounter a practitioner that is rushing through the visit with you, has poor bedside manner, is dismissive or inconsiderate about your feelings or concerns, voices limits to your progress due to personal or professional beliefs and understandings, has a pessimistic outlook, has narrow-minded thinking, etc.?*

Classroom training, textbooks, research, and documented science have their value as well as limitations. As practitioners, our greatest lessons and teachings, knowledge, and inspiration are gained through one-on-one interactions. It is imperative that we do not take these meaningful relationships for granted. It's imperative that we not discourage or dead-end our patients; instead, be realistic but encouraging, leave a window open for possibilities, for the unknown, for the infinite, for the miracles that happen. This is my message for all who read and listen. At any point in our lives, any one of us who are working as practitioners could be in the same or similar situation as our patients—looking, grasping, and yearning to feel a sense of hope, confidence, and courage—looking for signs that things will get better. It makes a difference to know the people who come in to help you are people who consider and value your life as if it were their own. Keep in mind, the value of the exchange taking place. Your presence can make a difference. Your job is not just a job, you are not there to display an attitude of "just doing what you have to do" because it's your shift or "this work pays the bills." Instead, come in with the heart and the intention that this is someone's life, worthy of your attention and time. At any given moment you are with that individual, you are giving of yourself and also receiving from them . . . a lesson, an idea, or a heartfelt exchange of compassion and gratitude. Know that your influence is significant.

When you encounter negativity, you are not to take the attitudes and behaviors of your interactions personally, that is not the intention of the interaction or exchange. You are a facilitator, an observer so that you are able to provide the best care possible, diffuse a situation, and also be open to receiving a lesson or two from the interaction. You have to be able to objectively appreciate that this is not about you; it's about the process we all become a part of, the lessons we are to learn. Together, we must all go through, grow through, stretch through, and rise up to the challenges offered through these experiences.

As you interact and deliver patient care make it a point to provide the kind of care you would want for yourself, your family, or your friends. With your sincere intention, you can help maximize the therapeutic value and outcome of the session. Identify, *"What is the true potential of this individual? What are his or her strengths and weaknesses? What are the desired or anticipated goals?"* Take a moment to reflect on how you feel about what you do. What is your attitude or approach at work and with people?

"Service which is rendered without joy helps neither the servant nor the served. But all other pleasures and possessions pale into nothingness before service which is rendered in a spirit of joy."

~ Mohandas Gandhi

Smile NOW, and smile often, for all to see and feel! Your smile can make a difference. Live and spread the message, "You are worthy, your life has value, and you matter." Live this way in your immediate life, in your home, at work, at school, and when you are out and about in the world.

AN AUTHENTIC SMILE WARMS and ENGAGES THE HEART

The origin of an authentic smile is generated from the heart.

The "authenticity" of a smile is validated from the heart and through the heart.

At the heart of an authentic smile is a warm and caring energy that influences the environment—its energy radiates throughout its immediate environment—its energy can be felt up close or at a distance.

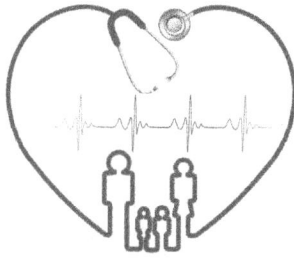

CHAPTER 5

INFLUENCES ON HEALTH AND WELL-BEING

STRESS, ANXIETY, PTSD

The effects of stress permeate every aspect of our lives. Stress has positive benefits to build us up and protect us and it also has adverse effects that can deplete our bodies and bring us down. The adverse effects are cumulative and over time, burden the body's defense system leading to illness and poor health. This outcome impacts our personal lives, workplace environments, and collectively our healthcare system. The financial costs are outrageous and perpetuate additional stress in an ongoing vicious cycle. An online *Forbes* article headline captured my attention,"Workplace Stress Responsible For Up To $190B In Annual U.S. Healthcare Costs."[1] This was quite alarming to read. It reported that at least 120,000 deaths per year have been linked to workplace stress with a significant factor being the lack of treatment due to people not having health insurance.

Stress is a natural part of life, however, there are harmful effects of ongoing high levels of stress such as workplace stress that is not new and does not get the attention it deserves. Adverse health effects from stress may include high blood pressure, depression, anxiety, pain, illness, over eating, or substance abuse.[1] Stressed employees miss work and are generally fatigued which make them prone to mistakes and injuries. This scenario can lead to decreased productivity, disability, and subsequent rise in health care costs

The biggest stressor and impact on our health and healthcare system is not having health insurance.[2] This factor contributes to both rising health care costs and mortality.

Additional sources of workplace stress include long hours, low wages, heavy workloads, lack of opportunity for growth and advancement, unrealistic job expectations, job insecurity, lack of control, work-family conflict, along with job pressures and demands from supervisors or employers which cumulatively take a toll on one's physical and mental health.[1,2]

I believe we can appreciate that the stress we feel is not isolated to one place or for one reason. When we talk about stress, it is a discussion about the varied and cumulative occurrences and the subsequent cumulative effects that if not adequately addressed lead us to disease and disastrous outcomes. If we are feeling stressed at home, we may take it into the workplace and if stressed at work, we take it home. In addition, we must consider other factors throughout the day that interplay with our stress responses and reactions. The overview by Health Advocate[3] provided a great reminder to consider caregiver stress — that caregiver stress significantly impacts work and family balance not only pertaining to raising children, but also with the added responsibility of caring for elderly parents. The challenge with balancing home and work life, and fitting in personal time requires deliberate and thoughtful attention to bring about effective strategies that can work for all involved. The complexity of developing a reasonable work-life model may be daunting but worthwhile.

The culture of the work environment matters. It affects the health and well-being of all individuals who work there and who transit through that environment. The way I view it, workplace stress affects everyone's bottom line which includes the employer's costs, the cost of individual health, and quality of life. We can spend a third to half of our day at work which consumes a good portion of our lives over time. Management expectations and practices should consider an integrated approach which takes into account the needs and desires of their employees to facilitate a healthy working relationship for the overall benefit to the organization and their employees. Incorporating stress management practices with rewards and incentives for small positive changes in the workplace can help foster employee job satisfaction and effectiveness with performance by improving morale and coping skills, reducing stress, and improving attention and focus to job tasks. Creating an environment where people feel valued, respected, trusted, are engaged in their work, don't fear losing their jobs, and have work hours that enable them to balance work and home life will prove to be more fulfilling and cost effective in the long run.

Surviving Stressful Experiences

Anger is a core piece of the natural survival response in human beings. It helps provide us energy to cope with life stressors. In cases of post-traumatic stress disorder (PTSD), any stress can have a person reacting as if his or her life was threatened. In PTSD, the tendency for being quick to anger, easily irritated, and impatience can significantly affect work and home life, and be linked to self-image and self-worth.

A study[4] on post-traumatic anger identified three key components: a higher more intense level of emotional and physical arousal and tension, aggressive responses to feeling threatened, thoughts and beliefs that there is threat all around even when this may not be true. The use of Cognitive-Behavioral Treatment (CBT) is a common treatment approach to help a person learn skills to relax and reduce tension, increase awareness to triggers and behavior patterns, and expand capacity for possible responses.[4] An important goal of treatment is to improve resilience and self-control. Self-monitoring exercises is another way to increase awareness to perceptions of threat which can help the person learn new ways of identifying and handling signs of emerging anger.

Veterans with PTSD often report difficultly with anger management.[5] Establishing and maintaining a positive therapeutic relationship between the Veteran and provider is of great importance to the course of treatment and outcome goals along with clarity from the provider for treatment expectations. Veterans with PTSD may also be dealing with depression, substance abuse, physical health problems and suffer with severe social and occupation impairments.[5] It is therefore very important the health provider assess for co-morbid conditions that may contribute to anger issues and compliance with therapy, and refer as appropriate

Stress management interventions are critical in helping to deal with anger problems and the heightened physiological responses.[4,5] Implementation of self-care practices, relaxation strategies, focused breathing, and social support become essential to defusing the anger response. Teaching strategies for effective communication is another valuable training to support the full course of treatment. The methods of active listening with the use of "I" statements, and creating awareness of the person's verbal and non-verbal communication help foster effective communication.[5] Veterans are provided psycho-education to better understand the constructs of anger and PTSD and to help develop skills for anger management. Therapeutic interventions are also offered in a safe, supportive group atmosphere where discussions and skill-building exercises are conducted.

Keep in mind there may be challenges to anger management intervention where the attempts to change may bump up against resistance. Consider that the person's anger and aggressive behavior may be a current source of self-esteem, or may be associated with distrust for authority figures, or if the person is a Veteran, the anger may have served a functional purpose while in a combat situation.[4,5] Any concerns and motivations should be discussed during the course of treatment.

Effects of Stress When Crisis Strikes

- *What happens when crisis strikes in your life, affecting you and your family's livelihood?*
- *When a life-altering crisis strikes, what do we do as practitioners, insurance companies, law enforcement, emergency response teams, patients, family, and friends?*
- *What do we do collectively as a community or a society?*
- *How do we react or respond in the midst of the situation?*
- *What actions, attitudes, behaviors, and support follow on into the long-term handling or management once the immediacy of the crisis is over?*

Initially, it is necessary and appropriate to react immediately, precisely, succinctly, and in a timely manner. Critical, life-saving measures are in the works, to stabilize and, ultimately, save lives. Emergency care is expedited to the greatest of our ability, utilizing resources to ensure the best outcome and recovery possible. Efforts are made to reduce further incident and to maximize functional outcomes.

During crisis, the sympathetic nervous system kicks in to assist and support both parties involved in this adrenalin rushing moment in time. Both the person or people providing life saving measures and the person or people receiving the care are in a high alert-high demand response. The autonomic nervous system is designed to automatically take charge in crisis.

- *What happens when the crisis is over?*
- *What happens to the nervous system that is left in a heightened, alert state?*
- *If this is your regular routine at work, how do you offset this?*
- *As for follow-on care, what do we do to help patients offset this heightened state, to account for this naturally occurring physi-ological response?*

The hierarchy of care works well to save lives, however, what is done to help manage the residual effects, the other issues that were not deemed "critical" during the initial phase of managing the crisis at hand?

The Autonomic Nervous System –
Parasympathetic and Sympathetic teeter totter:

Supply and Demand

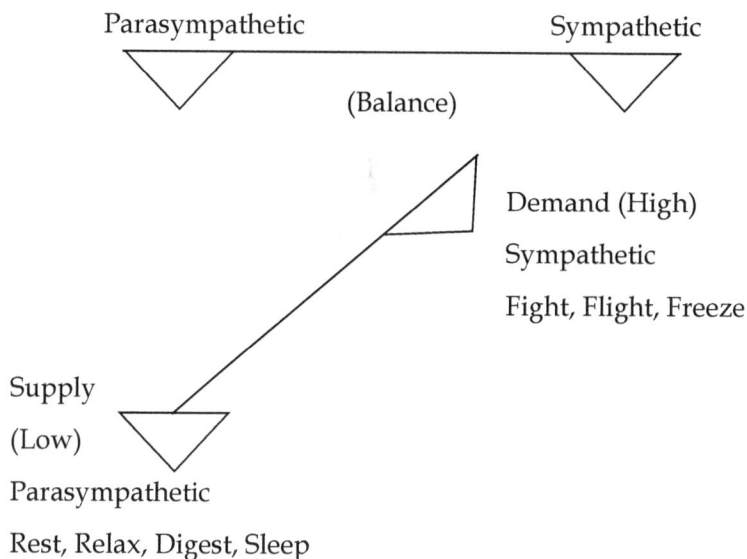

Parasympathetic   Sympathetic

(Balance)

Demand (High)

Sympathetic

Fight, Flight, Freeze

Supply

(Low)

Parasympathetic

Rest, Relax, Digest, Sleep

Supply and Demand

The body is a supply and demand system. The body does all it can to provide you what you need so that you can deal with the daily demands of your life. It strives to remain in balance (homeo-stasis) until the demand outweighs the resources and you start to trend downward. This is due to the lack of replenishment of nutrients to restock your supply. Think about having money in a bank account and all you do is withdraw from it. You may deposit a few dollars periodically, however, you may exceed what you have in the account and then you are now overdrawn and there is a penalty for that if you do not have overdraft protection. Or think about having a full tank of gas and you keep driving until you are now on "E", where the gas gauge is indicating EMPTY. That is a real bummer if you are not near a gas station!

COMPASSION FATIGUE

The American Institute of Stress defined compassion fatigue as, "The emotional residue or strain of exposure to working with those suffering from the consequences of traumatic events."[6] There are varying definitions and descriptions for compassion fatigue, however this definition resonated with me because of the word "residue", which refers to what is "left over" after all is said and done. You may enjoy your work and feel a sense of purpose and gratification as you engage day after day helping others, however, despite starting out with wonderful intentions, your ability to care and feel the same level of enthusiasm diminishes because you have taken on and taken home the side-effects from the varied experiences of those you have been caring for. Gradually over a period of time, your level of energy may slowly deplete, as if it erodes away…you may not feel like yourself anymore and may find yourself feeling emotionally and physically exhausted. This scenario is a process I am personally familiar with. As mentioned in the 2010 issue of the journal, *Best Practices in Mental Health,* compassion fatigue can occur as a result of working directly with clients or patients who experience crisis and trauma, and also when working with mentally ill populations.[7] The term has been used interchangeably with secondary trauma and vicarious trauma, however, distinctions can be made amongst these conditions. Compassion fatigue tends to develop over time, whereas secondary and vicarious traumatic stress can have a more immediate effect.

- *Is your inner world in need of quieting?*
- *Would you agree that you may not be as patient, friendly, or able to give your best when you are tired, frustrated, sick, worried, feeling overwhelmed, pressured, rushed, or burnt out?*

Your health and well-being can be at risk when you are continuously feeling over-stimulated and bombarded by your usual daily interactions at work and at home. Behind the scenes automatically operating on your behalf is your autonomic nervous system (ANS) responding to physiologically support all of your interactions which include responses or reactions to people, situations, pressures, demands, relationships external to you as well as the inner landscape of mind chatter, emotions, and sensations that may emerge or be suppressed in your body. Self-care can be seen as a preventive measure to help minimize the effects of compassion fatigue and support your care giving efforts. The importance of self-care is to lend support to a body that is striving to do the best it can. The body is a supply and demand system so resources can become depleted over time if there is no refilling or replenishing on a daily basis. Self-care practices should ideally support the physiological demand relevant to a specific diagnosis, daily choices, requirements, expectations, and take into account unknown factors.

Everything we do in life involves energy. As caregivers, the use of our physical, emotional and mental energy is required to support the person or situation we are caring for and sustain our personal efforts to care for ourselves at the same time. From personal experiences, observations, and review of this subject matter, the amount of energy expenditure can vary depending on many variables:

- Our attitudes and perspectives regarding the person or situation we are involved to care or look out for
- The length of time involved
- Type and quality of exposure
- Frequency of involvement or demand
- Whether involvement is direct or indirect
- The physical, emotional, mental severity or specific needs of the person being cared for and requirements of the

situation
- If there are others who share in the support
- Attitudes and perspectives of others able to positively or negatively influence person or situation
- Caregiver personal self-care habits

Creating awareness and implementation of prevention strategies for individuals and organizations at risk for trauma related conditions and burn-out can help to identify, address, and offset the potential of costly and damaging adverse health effects. The complexity of being a caregiver or being in a helping profession has far reaching effects that may go unspoken and often unnoticed until the health crisis is upon us. A person may start out feeling good and positive and then feelings subtly start to change, and the effects start to set in. Some of these effects may include depression, anxiety, grief, detachment, nightmares, sleep disturbances, physical ailments, problems with relationships, and compassion fatigue.

During the course of caring for others we may be witnessing suffering from a myriad of very sad, sudden, and traumatic events, while continuously listening to stressful and heart breaking stories, and intimately bonding and connecting through physical contact and similar experiences that are emotionally triggering. What was once positive in a desire to help can have negative and deleterious effects on our attitudes and performance, and become impactful on our energy expenditure. There are risk factors associated with providing services to vulnerable populations. As caregivers, at various levels during our daily interactions, we can be exposed to a variety of stressful and traumatic events and with repetition, time, and intensity secondary and vicarious traumatic effects can occur even with the best of intentions contributing to compassion fatigue.

Empathy and Compassion Fatigue with Human Connection...Choice, Reality, and Meaning:

As part of our human experience, we tend to vicariously live through the stories we hear and the scenes we witness, and often feel the thrill and joy alongside the pain and heartache...

We can hold on or let go of fear and suffering through bonds of love and connection...

We get to dream and hope with the people we care for, and get to feel inspired and uplifted when one triumphs over challenges or dies for a cause ...

Personal and organizational awareness and responsibility are required to manage and prevent compassion fatigue and burn-out. Daily practices and interventions are required to help offset the physical, emotional, and mental demands of care-giving. The mind-set and culture to support well-being and resilience requires communication, commitment, and community involvement. It is a shift in thinking to design wellness as the healthcare model rather than the current disease model which drives our costs up and burdens our system.

- *How would you rate your life satisfaction?*
- *What stressors are affecting you?*

Health professionals, people in healing professions, and caregivers can derive great satisfaction from providing compassionate and empathic care to others but not without risk of compassion fatigue. To achieve a sense of balance to this human desire and art of giving our time, energy, love and attention while working on sustaining our health and life-giving efforts requires deliberate and consistent attention to support our personal and professional quality of life. Health promotion and training on self-care practices should start early in our foundational education and continue as ongoing education and promotion in schools and work environments. Additionally, a positive win-win contribution in support of achieving work-life balance can be cultivated when our work environments recognize and appreciate the relationship between personal quality of life and professional quality of life by the standards they establish to support a healthy, thriving work environment.

POWERFUL HABITS

The things you say, do, and think repeatedly or automatically, whether good or bad, are considered habits. If you are not careful, habitual tendencies and patterns of behavior will run or ruin your life. Habitual patterns gradually work their way into your life through environmental and social conditioning, whether consciously or subconsciously. Many of your habits are learned through casual observation of behaviors repeated over a period of time. This "osmosis" type of learning is happening without your recognition of it. It is not until there is a problem or until you make a conscious effort to pay closer attention to your habitual behaviors that you begin to take notice of just what you are doing and why you are doing it. This "conscious" realization is how you begin to get to the root of your conditioning.

Your habits are activated automatically, a sort of underlying personal philosophy you create unintentionally, a philosophy that tends to run your life. This can be good if a habit is positive. If a habit is positive and life enhancing, it will work in your favor lending to your growth and success. However, if a habit is negative or unproductive, it will work against you, lending itself to procrastination, self-defeat, and stagnation.

What It Takes to Change Undesirable Habits: Two Vital Components

First Component: Changing an undesirable habit requires you have a meaningful, motivating WHY to sustain your efforts. This "why" will support your **decision** to change your habit, support the **commitment** you make to yourself and/or others, and will support the **disciplined action** you will take on a daily basis.

Second Component: Changing an undesirable habit requires a Replacement Behavior for the one habit you intend to change. You must replace the undesired habit with a more desirable behavior and then repeat consistently for a period of time, until it becomes a habit. It is not sufficient to just set out to stop a bad habit. You must substitute in a new and improved behavior until it becomes a new desired habit. Give yourself at least 30 days to instill your new habits into your life. This allows your nervous system to recondition and reorganize itself to a new program.

Living High On Life While Under the Influence

- *How many of you know how it feels to have a warm fuzzy feeling, a buzz, a feeling of having the edge taken off a bit from a couple glasses of wine, or a drink or two?*
- *How many of you know the feeling of invincibility and vulnerability that can occur as a result of alcohol or other substances floating throughout your blood steam, a subtle intoxication?*

Taking it further, how many of you know what it is to escape, lose your memory, or blackout from excessive levels of chemical substances in your blood stream?

- *How many of you smoke or get "high" because it makes you feel good or it relaxes you?*
- *Why do you do this?*

- *Why do you participate in these behaviors?*
- *What benefit do you derive from this?*
- *What if you could have this same feeling without these chemical substances?*
- *What if you could reach a point in your life where you felt fully engaged in life, felt excited and intrigued by what you could do and experience at your deepest level... a level that has your guard down, your senses more in tune to infinite possibilities, your heart open and available to risk and reveal, receive and restore – to feel like you always want to keep this feeling going because you feel more like your real self, you are at home in your heart, and you are at peace?*
- *Would this interest you?*
- *How would this change your life?*

Many people choose chemical substances to escape reality and avoid their true feelings. What benefit does this way of living really have, what do you gain in the long run? As with anything in life, extremes in any behavior are not the answer, but finding a relevant balance in your life is helpful. When you choose to engage in risky and illicit behaviors, you are also choosing to lose all perspective, choosing to lose self-control, and choosing to dismiss conscious judgment and awareness that could save you from making life altering mistakes.

As a physical therapist working in an acute care rehabilitation facility, I have seen firsthand the drastic, life changing outcomes of these mistakes. Working with people who become paralyzed after they have sustained head injuries and spinal cord injuries keeps me fully aware and appreciative of my blessings and opportunities.

I ask you to make a decision to change your life without the prompting and forceful awakening from tragedy. Let's not wait till "after the fact." Consciously design your life.

You are born with full potential to realize your passion and purpose. You are already fully equipped with everything to achieve your greatest desire. Commit to your personal growth, expand your awareness, befriend yourself, and be gentle and patient with yourself as you are changing and restructuring your life. Seek to balance all areas in your life. Get out and participate in activities that you enjoy doing and meet people who will support you as you are making positive changes in your life.

Surround yourself with people who believe in you and who challenge you!

Create your personal support team. If you don't have anyone in your immediate environment, connect with others through live events, organizations, groups, clubs, or outdoor activities, as well as watch, read, and listen to inspiring stories, etc. Continue to educate yourself, get to know and love yourself. Self-respect and self-discipline help to empower and build self-confidence. Commit to the growth and success of yourself and others through service and contribution. Life is full of amazing opportunities and infinite possibilities. Choose to get high on life!

PROCRASTINATION
Thoughts on Procrastination

- *Why do we put things off? Why do we wait for the last minute to get things done?*

I was once told that procrastination was a sign of self-confidence. I believed that for a while but then my view started to change. We are conditioned into a way of thinking and living. On a deeper level, my view is now that procrastination can be a form of avoidance, self-denial, a temporary confidence booster, a way to derive a sense of control, or an underlying addiction to the chemicals your body secretes as you rush to get things done. As a procrastinator, you give yourself an out to not fully engage yourself in life, to not grow and fully realize all of your talents and abilities, to not maximize on your full potential. Procrastination has some or all of these components built in: fear, complacency, lack of focus, disinterest, laziness, judgment, and false truths. You give yourself a "legitimate" excuse for why you are not further ahead in your life, for not fully being all you can be.

- *Is procrastination a factor in your life?*
- *How much more could you accomplish if you didn't procrastinate?*

It is a pleasure-pain cycle of behavior that you get caught up in. The temporary heightened state of pleasure or relief eventually works its way into a habitual pattern of procrastinating behavior which then becomes a way of life. This type of lifestyle does not allow you to maximize on your life, on what you could gain and what you could offer. Consider where you are at this time in your life and if procrastination is playing as a habit pattern in your life.

POSITIVE WORK CULTURES

We spend much of our waking hours at work in order to support our families and our lifestyles. Many people are struggling to meet personal and professional demands because of the ever evolving changes and challenges to really balance how we use our time and energy which are precious resources. We work to help effect the quality of our lives and the lives we serve.

- *What price are we paying for such noble sacrifices?*
- *What is the impact on our health and performance, on our relationships and livelihood?*

Many organizations have been working on various options for supporting employees such as working from home, flextime, and encouraging fitness and wellness in the workplace, however, when we consider the extensive amount of time spent at work it is also important to consider the environmental influences that affect well-being and impact outcomes. These outcomes are performance, health and relationships.

Well-being is fostered by a positive and engaged work culture.[8] The characteristics and values of leadership help set the tone within an organization and impact work culture and organizational effectiveness. The attributes of an effective leader include qualities of gratitude, kindness, empathy, trustworthiness, generosity, and a genuine concern for self and others.[8] These qualities for effective leadership apply to both the organization and the individual self-leader. Principles and practices of a positive work culture are where people inspire each other at work, derive a sense of gratitude and meaning from the work, treat others with respect and dignity, feel safe to express feelings and concerns or ask for help, and have regard for personal and social responsibility.[8] These qualities help foster commitment and engagement which can subsequently lead to authentic connections, innovation and empowerment, enhanced health and well-being, team resilience, and improved performance, productivity, and customer satisfaction.

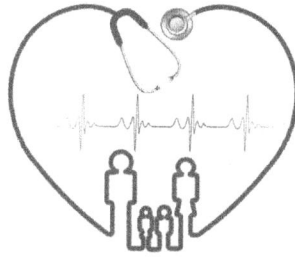

CHAPTER 6

INTRINSIC INFLUENCES ON CHANGE

VIEW ON CHANGE
The Influence of Thoughts and Voices in Your Head
We live in our heads most of the day.

- *What predominant thoughts are replaying over and over throughout our day?*
- *What thoughts are we manifesting into our reality, living out; what are we attracting to ourselves because of our thinking?*
- *Who and What are we listening to?*
- *How do we handle change, cope with change, respond to change, or deal with change in our personal lives?*

In order to see how change is regarded on a larger scale, we must view change from the individual's perspective. This goes back to familiarity. Change can be intentional, change can occur without choice, change can occur due to circumstances, and change naturally occurs with time and with aging. Although we know change is necessary for us to grow and improve the quality of our lives, we may be frightened of change. We want to know the effort is worth it. We want to know the outcome in advance — the unknown and the uncertainty may be so unsettling that we may not feel the effort to open ourselves to change is worth committing to and following through the process of change.

Change can be scary, yet it can be beneficial. It can be an opportunity that opens us up to possibilities that we never knew were available to us. Once we recognize how we handle change, we can then identify the types of influences that contributed to our coping ability. We know that our parents, teachers, and people in our immediate environment significantly influence our lives . . . *what then are we teaching our children?* Demonstrated actions, inactions, coping styles, and ease or difficulty with handling uncomfortable situations are lessons taught and learned by observation. This model is an impactful form of non-verbal communication. It is important to be mindful of the possible effects of our own behaviors and what we may be communicating to those around us, especially the lessons we are teaching our children. As parents and roles models, we want our children to learn effective coping strategies that will lend to their success in school, in relationships, in business, and in life.

- *How do we handle change collectively as a community and as a society?*

The awareness and consideration of our individual lives must come into play when we look at the bigger picture of change and the influences involved. We need effective leadership, mentorship, and support to bring about positive life-enhancing change; however, when the people we have in positions of influence exhibit poor behaviors and ineffective coping skills, they are not the best role models to lead or support effective, positive change.

This presents a challenge on a larger scale, to a very natural and necessary process for growth.

To facilitate positive and effective change requires that you are open, resilient, and objective — able to empathize, appreciate, persevere, provide constructive feedback, pause, and assess without hasty reacting with judgment, criticism, and blame as your first line of defense. Change is a constant in life, and unless you have these skills as mentioned, the challenge to change becomes an issue.

Change is essential to growth and an absolute in life...for everything is constantly changing whether you are aware of it or not, want it or not, can deal with it or not, or accept it or not. Change can be positive and it can be negative; it can feel good and not so good. The desire for change to feel good is a natural desire, but unrealistic. Change for healing and personal growth is many times out of your comfort zone, into the zone of uncertainty. This can be a challenge for many, especially if change arises out of life and death situations, traumatic incidents, relationship changes, childbirth, and many other circumstances that force you into change or subtly facilitate change. Realize that most of the time the process of change is not comfortable, it is simply necessary and you will grow as you go through it. Ultimately, it is all good.

CHALLENGE TO CHANGE

- *How many of us openly and readily welcome change into our lives?*

Often times we are resisting or dreading change. Through my own challenges with change and as a result of assisting others through their life changes, I have discovered that the sense of preparation is at the heart of effectively dealing with change. The anticipation of change happening and not being ready, willing or able to cope is a reality we face every day. Our beliefs and perspectives influence what we feel we can handle or are willing to consider in the face of uncertainty or crisis. It makes for a heart opening conversation and quick trip to one's bottom line of what really matters when I speak to people about life from an end of life perspective or from the perspective of life changing radically from what they have known. I have heart to heart discussions with my patients who are in the midst of dealing with a new diagnosis, a life-altering accident or injury, or possibly contemplating what should be their next step. I see a desire for a level of certainty which offers peace of mind and heart. What is really important to recognize about any decision we intend to make is to make it with knowing there are no guarantees, and that detaching from the outcome is where we will discover peace. Straddling the fence of faith and fear, trying to control outcomes or control the feelings or behaviors of others, invites frustration and anxiousness, stress and distress, and even anger and bitterness.

Can People Change?

I heard this question asked on television. My answer is YES! Change starts with an awareness that change is required or necessary, a desire to have, do or feel different, followed by a decision to change, then a commitment to yourself and the process. After these initial steps, you will then delve into a deeper awareness, an awareness that may find you feeling uncomfortable with yourself, others, or a situation. This may include a sense of uncertainty and flux. You may find yourself going through a myriad of emotions and feelings you may have never felt before or maybe had started to feel but put aside, denied, suppressed, and moved on with your life. When you reckon with deep-seated and unresolved emotions, this lends to your awakening, awakening to your deepest and authentic self. You get up close and personal with your fears and insecurities, your beliefs and attitudes, and your flaws and inadequacies. You start to take inventory of your choices and your decisions to this point in your life. You confront disappointment, despair, betrayal, denial, and remorse focusing in on yourself and your role that may have possibly enabled these emotions.

Ask yourself these few questions without judgment, blame, or shame:

- *What still challenges me today?*
- *Is there anything positive for me to learn or receive from my experiences?*
- *Is there anything positive I can share or teach from the lessons I have learned in my life?*

Remember, change is the only constant in life. You must accept it, welcome it, and grow with it. Changing your habits and behaviors may begin on the inside but recognize it has direct effects on both your inside and outside world. The practice of self-forgiveness, self-empathy, self-love, and patience are requirements for positive, healthy, and purposeful change. With greater self-awareness and self-care, you can then reach out into your environment as facilitators and contributors to effect positive change. The process of change is equivalent to the planting and nurturing of seeds for harvest. These seeds take root, grow, and sprout into a new, healthier perspective on life.

RESISTANCE TO CHANGE
A Mechanism for Coping, Controlling, and Asserting

Resistance to change comes from deeply rooted fears, insecurities, and anxieties, usually stemming from experiences in our early, formative years or influences from close, intimate relationships. The memories of experiences harbored deep within our cellular memory, memories that were chaotic, disruptive, traumatic, violent, or abusive can destroy our sense of wholeness and worthiness and render us defenseless and powerless. The act of resisting provides a barrier to block or avoid a memory or memories of a painful history. Resistance becomes the glue in which we are able to hold our sense of self and our life together; it's the anchor that keeps us steadfast, fixed in our ways, limiting our risks of uncertainty, seemingly helping us to remain "on course."

Resistance limits our openness and can fuel narrow-minded opinions. The repetitive practice of self-limiting viewpoints, and the ever present fearful reality of falling apart, reinforces a narrow window for receptiveness to change. Resistance may also show in perfectionistic behaviors as we stay on the continual cycle of striving for that perfect and certain outcome still beyond our reach. It is just a matter of time before change is recognized as being necessary to move forward; when life's outcomes are not what we desire; when the desire for happiness and purpose outweighs the hiding of one's pain and remorse from past experiences. There is an undercurrent to the resistance, an underlying fear of some sort. In order to change and move through fear, you have to face it. Make a list of your fears, then next to each one, write a possible benefit to overcoming every fear you have listed. Keep this in mind, we are all perfectly imperfect. It is time for you to move on, to step up, and to be in your power.

- *What could you gain from moving through your fear?*

Within every adversity lies a solution or a lesson. Seek to find it. In the midst of chaos and confusion you can find clarity and confirmation; recognize there is a message lurking within your "mess." Be brave, take heart, and dig deep—find the courage to turn your tragedy into a triumph.

> Use the energy you've been giving to resistance to keep you stuck, overwhelmed, and afraid to now move you up, out, and forward.

"I learned that courage was not the absence of fear, but the triumph over it. The brave man is not he who does not feel afraid, but he who conquers that fear."

~ Nelson Mandela

MOTIVATION FOR CHANGE

There are models that work as effective tools to help us initiate and promote behavioral change. The effective use of education, listening, and persuasion can help move our patients / clients towards action.

Theoretical Model of Change[1(p.224-225)]
- Precontemplation
- Contemplation
- Preparation
- Action
- Maintenance

Health Belief Model Concepts[1(p.222),2]
- Perceived Susceptibility / Threat
- Perceived Severity

- Perceived Benefits
- Perceived Barriers
- Cue to Action
- Perceived Self-Efficacy – The belief in being able to make the desired change is the most important. This is supported by increasing self-confidence and setting small, attainable goals.

Five A's Behavioral Intervention Protocol[1(p.222-223)]
- Address the issue
- Assess the patient
- Advise the patient
- Assist the patient
- Arrange for follow-up

As I think about my experiences in the acute inpatient rehab environment, the Theoretical Model of Change, the Health Belief Model, the Five A's Behavioral Intervention Protocol, and Motivational Interviewing (MI) all come together like a symphony orchestra. There is dynamic interplay as we seek to assess and identify where a patient truly is in his/her recovery process or readiness for change. From what I have experienced, I believe that many of our patients enter acute inpatient rehab in the Contemplation phase.[1] At this point in time, something has happened that may have forced change in their lives and they have a decision to make in moving forward. They are actively thinking and usually open to learning about how they can improve their health and regain their independence. Motivational Interviewing is an effective skill that can be developed with ongoing practice. The clinical use of MI helps activate the patient's own motivation for change and adherence to treatment.

The challenges and frustrations in healthcare that can often peak at times frequently remind me of the necessity of reflection.

I share an experience as an example of how we can assess, facilitate, or inhibit behavior change with our patients and clients. I
worked with a patient who had significant medical challenges
and there were concerns amongst the staff that she may have been
drug seeking. She tended to refuse many therapy sessions due to
generalized pain which she complained was not being managed
well. On my first visit with her I utilized the 5 A's to get to know
her. I was able to identify barriers, fears, and genuine desires and
goals. She showed me a picture of herself at a younger age. She
told me it was a positive reminder for a time in her life when she
felt good about herself. This picture was also a reminder of when
her mother made a comment to her that really hurt her feelings.
She shared a lot with me about her life going back to childhood
experiences. I had gained her trust and confidence. During this
session, I was able to guide her through a brief mindful practice.
All was well for that day. The next visit, she expressed that she
looked forward to working with me. She had walked more than
she had ever walked before with any therapy session. During this
time, she had further opened up to me about her adult child and
his challenges with care-giving responsibilities for a few family
members. She wanted more for him beyond his care-giving role.
She engaged in deeper discussions about her life. All was going
well for that day.

A couple days had gone by until our next visit which was a
totally different scenario. Her son was present and she was without the ability she had a couple days prior. She did not want to
get up, stated that she was unable to get up and I knew this was
a pattern of behavior throughout her stay experienced by other
therapists. The dynamics had changed with her son's presence. I
did my best to encourage participation and reminded her of how
capable she was but this only led to her feeling that it was my
interests versus her interests. I was now perceived as a threat. I
tried to make amends later but she wanted nothing more from

me. I felt very frustrated and sad and later recognized that I should have stopped way sooner in the conversation.

After personal reflection, denial was in play for her. I recognized the forces that affected this undesired outcome. There was a level of high emotion with her son being present which provided attention as well as distraction, and lent to evoking past experiences and patterns which included her sense of low self-esteem and low-self-efficacy. She had reverted back to pre-contemplation.[1] I also recognized that I was not as empathetic as I could have been yet really wanted her to continue what she had begun. What I am reminded and am grateful for with this topic of behavioral change is that as practitioners, our own passions and desires for our patients can get in the way of listening objectively, may trigger the "righting reflex"[3(p.7)] and then we miss the opportunity to elicit the patient's own motivations for change.

Intrinsic Factors

- *What moves you to do anything or nothing at all?*

Within you is the power to change. The awareness you have around the choices you make and the behaviors you engage in are the starting point. Recognizing your habits, even the most insignificant or smallest of habits that you may think do not have that much affect on your health and well-being, if done regularly has an ever-mounting cumulative effect on your health and the quality of your life.

SELF-REFLECTION QUESTIONS:

How would you <u>Describe</u> Healthy?

Does being healthy matter to you?

What would it mean to you to be healthy?

How does your health affect your relationships?

What would it mean to your relationships to be healthy?

How would your life change if you had problems with your health?

What factors influence or affect your health?

How do you define inspiration?

Is there anything that inspires you?

How do you define motivation?

Is there anything that motivates you?

On the number line, where do you feel you are right now with your health?
Estimate: Poor=0-3 Fair=4-5 Good=6-8 Great=9-10

(Poor) ← 1 − 2 − 3 − 4 − 5 − 6 − 7 − 8 − 9 − 10 → (Great)

Your daily choices add up either way. Based on your answer, what action or inaction could you do within the next 24 hours that could raise your number towards great or lower your number towards poor? Give an answer for each direction.

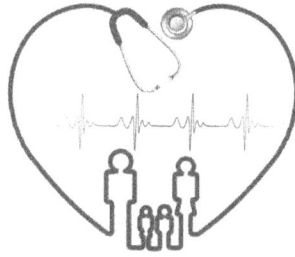

CHAPTER 7

SELF-CARE MANAGEMENT

PREVENTIVE HEALTH AND CHRONIC CARE

Building the Case for Chronic Disease Prevention Through Self-Care Management

There are numerous behavioral factors associated with the development of chronic illnesses. Public education and health promotion are critical and effective components, interventions, and strategies for prevention and management of chronic diseases. From early childhood, we establish habits and patterns of behavior and make lifestyle choices that affect our current and future health. The motivation for change typically occurs after a significant life-altering event. Health care promotion through self-care management can be a useful and practical approach in motivating people to adjust behaviors and lifestyles.

The prevalence and desired control for cardiovascular disease is a major public health challenge in the United States. Risk factors for cardiovascular disease include diabetes, high blood pressure, high total cholesterol, smoking, and obesity. The American Heart Association® report[1] stated that the presence of one major risk factor at age 50 was associated with an increased lifetime risk for cardiovascular disease. In a relevant study,[2] the prediction of low lifetime risk for cardiovascular disease was associated with the absence of cardiovascular risk factors at age 50. These reports[1,2] proposed that early intervention and prevention efforts that focus on healthy lifestyle choices and modifications can prevent the development of cardiovascular risk factors.

Daily self-care behaviors and lifestyle habits are critical elements for preventative health care as well as disease management. It is important to consider how people cope with their illness and how they deal with stress and emotions that affect their well-being. According to Greaves and Campbell, "Changing the self-care behavior of patients is relevant not only for preventing future health problems, such as heart disease and lung cancer, but also in mediating the course of long-term conditions."[3(p.814)] This statement captures the broad spectrum importance that deliberate and strategic self-care practices and interventions can have on a person's health over the course of time.

Greaves and Campbell reported that many patients simply do not follow nutritional guidelines and do not participate in recommended levels of physical exercise or activity. They further identified that the patient's adherence to medications was at approximately 30-50% and it was estimated that around 75% of hospital admissions for diabetes and asthma could be avoided through acts of self-care.[3] There are many types of self-care interventions and strategies that are offered at different levels of intensity, are delivered in variety of settings, and can be disease specific. They can be delivered individually or in group format. Interventions include teaching patients coping strategies and helping them to design daily action plans. In addition, components that support effective self-care practices and behaviors include addressing patient motivations, barriers to change, emotional responses to illness, and involving family and social support.[3] Extended support from family, peers, health professionals, and community programs can help with implementation and lend to the long term success of healthy self-care practices.

Health professionals, particularly primary care providers can support, help increase awareness, and reinforce self-care interventions and practices. Ideally, there should be buy in from the entire health care team in order to develop an efficient system that supports effective approaches to self-care interventions. Additional efforts to coordinate, integrate, and reinforce the benefits of self-care, especially regarding illness prevention, can be provided through public health and community health promotion initiatives. Optimal care can be better achieved if we seek ways for patients and health professionals to work together, maximizing on each other's expertise.[3]

As stated in the findings by Ory et al[4] "National Study of Chronic Disease Self-Management," Americans 65 years and older are disproportionately affected by chronic illness with over 70% having at least two chronic conditions. The data revealed that when individuals increased their number of health conditions there was a direct correlation to adverse outcomes; a corresponding increase in poor functional ability, increase in unnecessary hospitalizations, adverse drug-related situations, conflicting medical advice, and duplication of tests, all of which contribute to higher health costs and greater financial outlay for government programs such as Medicaid and Medicare.

The National Council on Aging (NCOA) reported[5] that:
- Approximately 80% of older adults have one chronic disease.
- 68.4% of Medicare beneficiaries have two or more chronic diseases.
- 36.4% have at least four or greater chronic diseases.
- 95% of costs incurred by older Americans are due to chronic diseases.

According to the National Council on Aging, greater than two-thirds of funds spent on our nation's health care are for chronic disease and less than 1% of fiscal resources are spent on prevention efforts to improve overall health.[5]

In order to address these conditions, new strategies are required that focus to improve function and delay deterioration, and should also recognize the problems people face in their daily lives.[5] There is a growing interest in self-management programs that focus on patient empowerment and control for the management of their health conditions. A well recognized and researched program is Stanford University's Chronic Disease Self-Management Program (CDSMP).[4-10] The CDSMP program is a low-cost program that has online and in-person components. The live workshop is led by two trained facilitators, with one or both facilitators having at least one chronic illness. The program runs for a 6-week period, once a week for 2.5 hours per session and teaches participants the skills they require to effectively manage their health conditions as they concurrently receive peer mediated support through sharing of experiences. The workshops are offered in a variety of community based settings and common topics include nutrition, exercise, pain management, handling emotions, problem solving, goal setting, action planning, and communicating with their health practitioners. The effectiveness of the CDSMP has been considered significant due to measurable health and cost savings benefits.[7-9]

The reported outcomes at six month and twelve month follow-ups revealed a reduction in emergency room visits and hospitalizations. The demonstrated success of the CDSMP validates that such evidenced based programs increase physical activity and health outcomes, offer health and life-enhancing strategies and cost saving benefits, however, support to increase awareness and integrate and deliver these programs require that we strengthen collaborative efforts amongst healthcare practitioners and organizations, community partnerships, and public health agencies.[7-9]

Self-management programs can help to optimize successful health outcomes. A key component to any successful self-management program is to identify early on any reported barriers or potential barriers by participants.[11] Barriers can be numerous... they may include financial or transportation constraints, insurance issues, lack of awareness of resources, adverse health effects of disease process, lack of understanding the effects of medication, lack of social or medical support – low level of confidence, depression, feelings of overwhelm, low health literacy, debility, and more.[11] These barriers can interfere with the self-management process and outcomes. The relevance of a subjective history as it relates to subjective outcomes is of great importance, especially for seniors with multi-morbidities. As stated in the study by Bayliss and Colleagues, "A lower perceived health status is predictive of mortality, and low levels of physical functioning predict mortality and functional dependence."[11(p.396)] The study added that the low level of physical functioning was predictive of increased utility of healthcare resources.[11(p.398)]

Bandura stated, "Self-Management is good medicine."[12(p.245)] He also stated that it is important to have a broader more expanded perspective on health promoting practices that will encourage participation and hence the collective efforts of practitioners from various disciplines. The quality of one's health is significantly influenced by lifestyle habits and therefore health promotion efforts should begin with setting goals and not necessarily the means to the goals.[12] Health habits require more than willpower to change current practices. Self-management requires self-motivating incentives, self-regulatory skills, and social support to sustain the life and health-enhancing practices. It is noteworthy that people at greatest risk tend to ignore preventive or remedial health services and resist seeking assistance, however, according to Bandura, this population responded better to online guidance with use of the Internet because it was readily accessible, convenient, and offered a sense of anonymity. He also added that goal adoption can set the stage for self-directed change and self-efficacy beliefs become the predictor for the adoption of healthy practices.[12]

"Perceived self-efficacy to control thought processes is a key factor in regulating thought produced stress and depression."[12(p.133)]

"Efficacy beliefs influence how people feel, think, motivate themselves, and behave."[13(p.118)]

According to Social Cognitive Theory, the core determinants for successful health promotion and disease prevention involve knowledge of health benefits and risks, perceived self-efficacy that one has control over personal habits and practices, outcome expectations about benefits and costs regarding modified health habits, specific health related goals that one sets along with specific plans and strategies for realizing them, and perceived facilitators involved as well as structural and social impediments to the changes they desire.[14(144)] Personal goals are established from one's value system which sets the course direction and acts to reinforce personal commitment towards successful behavioral change. The highly valued goals should provide self-incentives and enhance motivation towards long-term health habit and personal change.

Self-efficacy influences patients' perspectives and behaviors. People tend to avoid what they feel incapable of accomplishing and pursue what they feel competent to perform. Long-term health prognosis is determined by a culmination of small daily behavioral choices that affects the direction of our health and our lives. A vigorous sense of efficacy lends to motivating and engaging participants in task performance; fueling effort and persistence towards mastering activities.[15] Self-efficacy scales can be designed for specific domains of functioning, are specific to a given population, and require the assessment of competencies and challenges that pertain to specific behaviors and situational context in which they take place.[15] The use of such measures can provide greater perspective to the role of perceived self-efficacy in modification and maintenance of health behaviors.

The focus on adolescent health for health promotion is a priority around the globe. This group is identified as being within the age range of 10 to 19 years.[16] Adolescence is a time of rapid development and transition where the child grows and shifts into adulthood. This is an influential period of time when the adolescent develops a sense of autonomy and independence from family through experimental behaviors and experiences. During this time, the efforts to establish identity, self and body image, and relationships directly influence health habits. It is an era of transformation through intense social, emotional, physical, cognitive, and hormonal changes and where customs and habits are established for a lifetime. The study, "Knowledge and Practices of Teenagers About Health,"[16] identified that when adolescents were asked for examples of who they considered healthy, their first response was examples of family members, then physical education teachers, and lastly friends. The data from this study also revealed that the adolescents' perspective of health was viewed as the absence of disease and that many of the adolescents did not consider themselves healthy although they expressed having knowledge of how to stay healthy.

Adolescents tend to seek immediate pleasure without regard for maintaining health. Social and cultural representations through family and media affect adolescent perspectives and subsequent choices and behaviors. Fashion standards established by external beauty models have effects on health habits and self-image as well as self-esteem and self-confidence. In efforts to bridge the gap between what adolescents know and what actions will help them adopt healthy habits and encourage self-care practices, the teenager's knowledge should be valued by the health professional and an exchange of knowledge should be take place in order to reach common ground.[16] This alliance and foundation works in favor to help create a therapeutic action proposal that can motivate and support the adolescent towards a more proactive role in their personal care.

Within the past two decades, children dealing with chronic conditions have doubled with an estimated increase from 13% to 27% and half to two thirds of children and adolescents with chronic conditions were significantly affected by non-adherence to treatment regimens.[17] The necessity to engage patients and families in self-management behaviors is a high priority. New health care policies are required that expand coverage to include reimbursement for self-management education programs and resources.

Four domains have been specified to influence self-management behaviors[17]: the individual, family, healthcare system, and community influences. Supportive social influences, especially during adolescence, can help teenagers make a developmental shift from exclusive parental influences to effective peer influences.[17] Children and adolescents' perception of social situations as it relates to engaging in vital self-management behaviors is a strong influence. The youth may feel embarrassed or self-conscious, fear any stigma, and not want to draw attention to their illness as a result of adhering to their treatment regimen. If these youth had appropriate peer support, this could promote adherence and reduce fears and embarrassment.

There are various online programs that offer educational, engaging, and interactive content for self-management training. Self-management promotion[17] is essential for the pediatric population to:

1. Promote access to preventive health resources
2. Provide education and support on disease management
3. Provide skills training to effectively cope with emotional and social pressures
4. Promote self-advocacy
5. Offer mentoring programs

For the adolescent population, the role of healthcare clinicians in self-management support is significant, especially as a mentor role model. The promotion of pediatric self-management requires a comprehensive approach to include advocacy from healthcare clinicians and health care policies. Healthcare providers can benefit from new and advanced trainings to help improve listening skills and collaborative goal setting. Coordinated self-management interventions can reduce preventable health care utilization and illness related morbidity and have significant impact on long-term health outcomes and health care costs.[17]

Explored self-management experiences for adolescents living with chronic health conditions have helped to identify the barriers to self-management and the challenges faced by youths to include risk factors for psychosocial problems, physical and psychological abuse and sexual exploitation. For adolescents with chronic health conditions, protective over-parenting was considered a possible hindrance to self-management and over-protection was identified as a predictor of future abuse in relationships for women with physical disabilities.[18] An important consideration for adolescents who are living with a chronic condition is their perspective on life. The importance of peer interaction and decreased focus on health behaviors and long-term effects of disease process is normal for this age group, however, ignoring protocols and not adhering to proper disease management can be detrimental for this vulnerable population.

Self-management strategies and skills training should provide a sense of meaning and purpose for the adolescent. Healthcare practitioners have an important role in helping to encourage negotiations regarding self-management.[16,18] Practitioners and health care facilities can derive community support from partnerships with organizations such as transitional care and independent living facilities which can be effective alliances that help foster positive, empowering behavioral experiences for the adolescent.

The regime for self-management and self-care is demanding and complex for adolescents with chronic health conditions, therefore creating an atmosphere that is engaging and conducive to learning can motivate and encourage positive, proactive health behaviors.[18,19] The distribution of responsibility will change over the developmental course of adolescence. The ultimate goal is for the adolescent to have a sense of autonomy within the context of parental / family support. For example, with chronic and complex conditions like spina bifida and diabetes, the adolescent can begin to transfer responsibility from parent to self, at least in taking on greater levels of responsibility as they get older.[18,19] The driver's license model best exemplifies the building of self-management, allowing the transition from "permit" to license, where monitoring and limitations are in place and graduated responsibility can be utilized for shared decision making in self-management.[18] For this young and complex population, shared responsibility between the parent and the adolescent offers the best outcomes.[19]

Implications of Self-Care Management in Clinical Practice

Self-care management encourages daily self-care behaviors and lifestyle habits that are critical elements for preventative health as well as disease management and can possibly prevent the development of cardiovascular risk factors. Healthcare practitioners are perceived as models and advocates for the healthcare system.[16,18] The health practitioner's role is influential along the lifespan continuum; from the initial planting of seeds via open dialogue to promote self-management to the follow-up and sustained efforts for long-term effectiveness and success of self-management implementation. Promotion and facilitation of self-care behaviors are influenced by the individual health practitioner's views, beliefs, and personal self-care practices. Self-efficacy plays a critical role and must be considered an integral part of patient or participant assessment. This also includes the beliefs of the practitioner, the perceived ability to provide the most appropriate and effective care to his/her patients. Perceived self-efficacy affects how one copes with situations. People are more vulnerable to stress and depression with a low sense of efficacy.[15] It is important to identify any internal and external barriers or challenges to health behaviors/performance as it relates to self-efficacy.[11,18] Assessment of barriers can be made through a combination of formal interviews and observations. Identifying specific task demands can help support patients in successful engagement and achievement of positive, healthful behavioral experiences and hopefully lead to mastering of health promoting behavioral activities.

Summary of Benefits to Self-Care Management

Beliefs and expectations play directly into health behaviors. An effective self-management program must recognize the powerful influence of perceived self-efficacy and social engagement, and the collaborative effort and support of family, peers, health practitioners, and community. Predictors of successful health outcomes start with the individual's baseline self-efficacy beliefs and are supported by the self-efficacy beliefs of the self-management program.[12]

> "Self-Efficacy beliefs shape the outcomes people expect their efforts to produce." Bandura[14(p. 145)]

It can be challenging to accurately measure self-efficacy, therefore valid and reliable measures of self-efficacy must take into account a broader perspective and understanding as it is important to identify competencies and specific challenges relevant to the diagnosis, social and environmental conditions and situations, as well as individual perspectives and beliefs surrounding all of it.[15]

Self-Management programs should teach appropriate disease management and self-care skills while integrating efficacy beliefs that will enable participants to manage emotional and social pressures that can influence their decisions and behaviors. Supporting and guiding people in their motivation to change requires appropriate resources and environmental and social support to realize and sustain those changes. Under the self-management model, people learn how to self-direct and monitor their health behavior, motivating and guiding their own behaviors and habits as they are their own agents of change.

Important considerations for the medium to deliver and evaluate self-management training and support include the participant's age, health condition, health literacy, and personal preference. Technological advancements, especially with the Internet, have provided a platform for interactive and engaging content delivery. This particular platform is a viable resource that can support healthy self-management behaviors, helping to motivate and engage the participant, foster adherence to healthy habits, and thereby enable participants to effectively manage their chronic health condition.[12,14] The online Internet option is often appealing to adolescents and high risk patients. A combination of in-person small group, peer mediated workshops and online access to interactive and engaging content has been shown to have positive health outcomes as evidenced in the CDSMP model.[4-10]

Health promotion must be adopted as a societal commitment, and be structured with incentives and resources to support healthful behaviors from early childhood and reinforced throughout the lifespan. Efforts with health education should be comprehensive and focus on prevention of illness as well as improving disease management through healthy lifestyle choices to include personal accountability and responsibility for desired outcomes. There are social and cultural influences across the lifespan which must be considered for any self-management intervention.

Implementation of self-care management practices is about choice and personal commitment to better care for oneself which can offset the development of cardiovascular risk factors and subsequent cardiovascular disease and a myriad of other preventable life-altering and debilitating illnesses. This understanding will not only affect the quality of life for the individual, but can have a rippling and profound impact on public health at local, state and global levels. The psychosocial-emotional and financial challenges faced by society can change and improve as the individual decides to take personal responsibility for making healthier choices on a daily basis. Bottom line, implementation of an effective self-care management practice provides a personal and practical course of action that is essential to healthy living, longevity, and productivity, and simultaneously provides a viable solution that can benefit society as a whole.

TUNE-IN
Interrelations of the Body System

The body is a dynamic, intuitive, and self-regulating system. All systems work together, exchanging information, interacting, compensating, and adapting throughout the day. An example below gives you a basic idea of the interdependency of the body system as it relates to achieving Optimal Health.

> **Your Communication System:**
> Mind
> Body
> Heart
> Spirit
> Emotions
>
> Inside of YOU is the POWER to CHANGE YOUR LIFE!

YOU CAN GROW STRONGER AND LIVE LONGER!

- *What does your body want and need to be Happy, Healthy, and Prosperous?*
- *What is your body communicating to you?*
- *What aren't you listening to?*
- *Why aren't you listening?*

Your Posture, Breath, and Attitude

- *What Do They Have In Common?*

The body is very good at adapting to what you ask of it. Postural or positional adaptations create restrictions and tension in the system. This leads to the body having to compensate due to affects on respiration, blood flow, movement, and function. Over a period of time, this may lead to musculoskeletal and neuromuscular imbalances contributing to pain, discomfort, and stress-related symptoms.

- *Are you aware of your posture, how you sit in your car, how you stand, how you walk?*
- *Are you aware of patterns and positions you hold yourself in, whether positions for leisure, work-related tasks, or positions for sleeping and eating?*
- *Are you aware of what your body is doing?*
- *Are you aware of your shoulders rising up to your ears?*
- *Are you bracing your body in some way right now?*
- *Are you aware that your hip is shifted to one side, as you sit or stand, leaning to one side or the other?*
- *Are you aware of your breathing while you are sitting in traffic, when you are busy at work, or standing in line waiting to check-out and things are taking too long?*
- *Are you aware of your body's behavior and habits at any given point in time during your day?*

Many of you are holding your breath throughout the day and don't realize it. Along with breath holding, you can find yourself clenching your teeth. Clenching teeth is a postural habit that will affect your attitude, your comfort, how you hold your shoulders, and it will affect blood flow and lymphatic flow through the neck.

FOCUS ON ABILITY

Within you is the power to create your life, to change your life, and to direct the course of your life! Recognize that your precious life source ENERGY is being used up by any self-doubt and self-defeating thoughts. Wherever your attention goes, so does your energy. You can choose to let fear sit in the driver's seat of your life, creating angst and anxiety and producing experiences that have you feeling helpless and out of control. You can focus on everything that is wrong and undesirable with your life, the flaws and imperfections of life, and your energy will be expended in that direction. What I feel confident in sharing from my own personal and professional experiences is that focusing on your ability, to whatever degree of ability, is the best use of your precious energy. Celebrating small successes helps build on greater successes. Your perspective, attitude, effort, and the quality of your breathing directly support your ability.

Recognize the Transformative Effects of Your PERCEPTION!
Decide to take full responsibility for your life.
Commit to living your best life possible.
Take Courageous Action in the direction you want to go.

Create Your Life:

1. *Decide to take full responsibility for your life, to control your energy.*
2. *Commit to your decision.*
3. *Visualize and Feel what you desire. (If you don't specifically know what you want, at least be clear on what you don't want.)*
4. *Acknowledge WHY you want it.*

Suggestions:
1. "QUIET" Yourself; "BE STILL"
   Connect with God and "Self," through Meditation or Prayer

Engage in the Daily Practice of Applied FAITH and GRATITUDE

Ask Your "Inner Guidance" for help, for direction, for peace . . .

2. SELF-REFLECT: Take Inventory of Your Life

3. OPEN your Mind and Heart to FORGIVENESS
    Take ACTION to FORGIVE Yourself and Forgive Others!
    LET GO of the ENERGY you give any Undesirable Experience to Control You!
    STOP Talking about IT!
    STOP REPEATING HISTORY!

4. MAKE A COMMITMENT TO YOURSELF
    - *What do you really want?*
    - *What don't you want?*

5. VISUALIZE and FEEL . . .
    Your Dreams
    Your Goals
    Your Heart's Desire

6. DECIDE to RESOLVE and EVOLVE
    ALIGN Your HEART and MIND with Your Decision

7. IMPLEMENTATION: Take DECISIVE and PURPOSEFUL ACTION STEPS!
    FOCUS your Attention
    - *What is your main focus for today?*
    - *Where do you want to direct your energy?*
    - *Where will you invest your valuable time, attention, and energy?*

8. DAILY Positive Self-Talk (in present tense affirmations) YIELD to Your "SPIRIT of WONDER and CREATIVITY" Make Room in your Heart for that which you DESIRE and DESERVE

You are Better Able to Hear or See Your Options and Truth when You . . .

"QUIET" YOURSELF. Seek inner wisdom.

BE OBJECTIVE... STEP OUTSIDE YOURSELF. BE IMPERSONAL.

Become an OBSERVER of your life and behavior.

GET TO KNOW YOUR "EGO."

Activity: Draw a Circle—Divide the circle into separate sections; each section represents the various areas of your life. Become the Observer: Position yourself outside of the circle looking in at the areas of your life—take a close, objective, impersonal look at what is inside the circle.

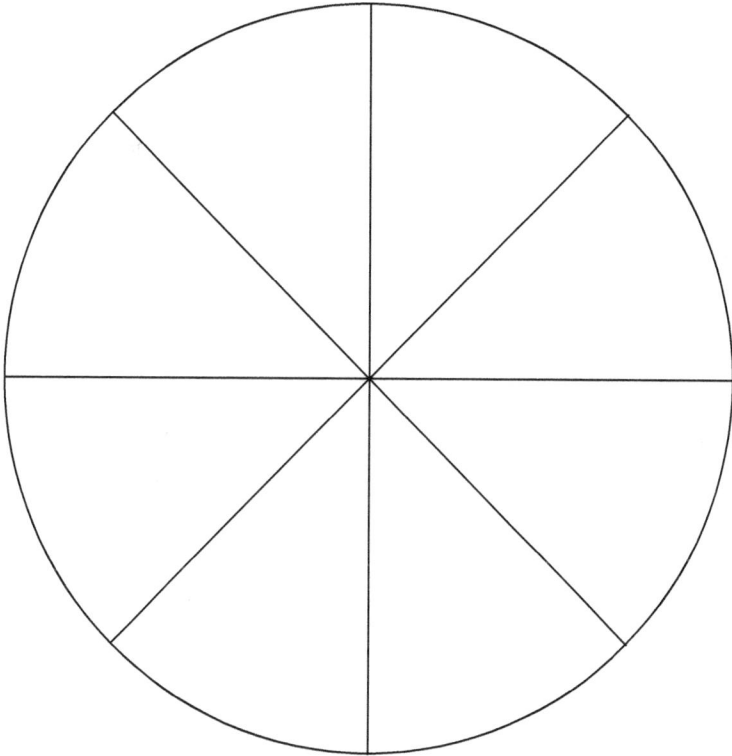

YOUR 'WHY' MATTERS
CREATE THE EXPECTATION:

- *What Is Your Heart's Desire for the Life You Have Been Granted?*
- *What is Your "WHY" for this Desire?*
- *What are Your Core Values?*

CORE VALUES:
- Core Values Guide Your Behaviors and Actions

1. Write a Personal Mission and Vision Statement for Your Life.
2. Write down Your GOALS: Be Realistic with Short-Term and Long-Term Timelines.
3. Prepare a Plan to Achieve Your Goals:
   Suggested Areas of Focus: Health, Personal Growth, Relationships, Finances, Lifestyle, Service, and Contribution

From Your Heart, Answer These Questions

- *Looking Ahead, What Would You Like to Accomplish in Your Lifetime?*
- *What Do You THINK You Deserve from Life?*
- *What Do You FEEL You Deserve from Life?*
- *Is there any difference or similarity between the two answers?*
- *WHO in Your Immediate NETWORK Supports Your DESIRES?*

Ask Yourself:

- *Do You DESIRE and DESERVE to be SUCCESSFUL?*
- *Do You DESIRE and DESERVE to REACH YOUR GOALS?*
- *Do You DESIRE and DESERVE LOVE in Your Life?*
- *Do You LOVE YOURSELF?*

MIND AND BODY AT EASE

Get Into Your Groove and Allow for Flow and Ease in Your Life

Get and Stay FOCUSED! Constantly work to develop and refine yourself. Do whatever it takes to make it happen. Allow yourself to be driven by passion and purpose. Embrace challenges no matter what they may be. It is important to remember the actions or inactions taken on a daily basis affect and change lives, starting with your own!

Tongue-Jaw-Neck Check:

Soften your tongue and jaw. Take a deep breath, in through your nose and out through your mouth, while maintaining your softened tongue. Tension will naturally release from your shoulders— they will drop into a position of ease. For that moment allow yourself to feel what you feel. With practice, you will sense a softening in your face, neck, throat, and chest. This exercise will help calm and quiet your body throughout your day. It will also promote a positive effect on your attitude as well as a deeper a sense of ease; ease with your breathing because a feeling of "flow" is taking place throughout your body.

Raising Daily Consciousness through Personal Awareness
RECOGNIZE:
1. Your Day consists of a Series of Small Choices, either Beneficial or Harmful.
2. The Little Things you do on a daily basis Add Up— Benefiting or Hurting you.
3. Every Encounter or Interaction is a Relationship; an Exchange of Ideas, Information, Feelings, Energy . . . an Opportunity . . .
4. You are either on the Path of Prevention or Manifestation of Disease.
5. You either Live with Faith or Fear.
6. What you Resist will Persist!
7. An Attitude of Gratitude helps you to Keep Things in Perspective

LANGUAGE FOR SUCCESS
The Business of Living a Healthy, Prosperous, and Abundant Life Requires You Use Language for Success
Your words matter! What you say matters!

- *How do you speak to yourself?*
- *How do you speak to others?*
- *What words do you use regularly to refer to tasks or activities?*
- *Do the words you use make you feel good?*

Make every day a great day whether it feels great or not. Reflect an attitude of gratitude every day in every way. Consider that when you use words like hard, try, or can't, your energy dips. Achieve a new outlook and attitude immediately by using words that lift, energize, and empower you.

Suggestions on new Key Words for your Daily Vocabulary:
Replace with New Empowering Key Words

Too Hard → Very Challenging

I will Try → I will do it, I commit to it

I Can't → I can, I will, I will do my best

IMPLEMENTATION OF CONSISTENT DAILY DISCIPLINES CAN HELP YOU SHIFT FROM:

ACTIVITY	→	PRODUCTIVITY
STAGNATION		GROWTH
PROCRASTINATION		COMMITMENT
FATIGUE		ENERGY
FRUSTRATION		INSPIRATION
BOREDOM		ENTHUSIASM
FEAR		FAITH
DISTRUST		TRUST
INSECURITY		CONFIDENCE
OVERWHELM		OVERFLOW
FRAGMENTED		WHOLENESS
DISTRESS		HARMONY
TURMOIL		PEACE

CULTIVATING COMPASSION AND EMPATHY

Self-Compassion

Compassion is an archway that opens to your heart's path for inner healing, resolving conflict, and restoring relationships. The interweaving of empathy and heartfelt intention for a positive, constructive and peaceful way forward complements the process of cultivating compassion. Imagine that once you step through this archway you are surrounded by the fresh air of appreciation and acceptance—feel the infusion of appreciation and acceptance gently permeating each and every cell, acknowledging all that you have been through.

Compassion offers you a perspective that expands your view of what is possible and expands your heart's capacity for self-love and forgiveness, as well as love and forgiveness of others and a healthier overall view of a situation or experience. You may weep along this path, deeply feeling your heart's desires for peace and serenity, and sensing harmony and genuine relief. Sincerely open to your feelings. Give yourself permission to feel whatever you feel, without judgment, aversion, resistance, blame or shame. Compassion helps you to be deeply present with your emotions, especially with painful and highly charged emotions like grief, anger or rage. Self-compassion is like welcoming in a close and trustworthy friend to sit with you, listen to you, allowing you to express what you feel, recognizing your sincere efforts, and acknowledging your pain and struggle. Your willingness and patience to simply be with your pain and suffering help you to cultivate compassion.

Compassion For Others

When we hold others on the hook for wrongdoing or hurtful behaviors, we are also holding ourselves on the hook. The process of allowing compassion to infuse into our cells and into our being cultivates an inner state of peace and tranquility. This is the environment that helps us make room for resolving deeply painful emotions. It does not condone or deny the behavior or action that caused the pain, it simply offers a space to rest peacefully with all of what we feel, and this helps to dissipate, dissolve, and take the "charge" off a highly charged emotion. This path simultaneously nurtures as it offers us a way to grow through our experiences and provides us another lens in which to view and renew from our most powerful and purest foundation...the Divine presence of unconditional love and acceptance of ourselves and life itself.

We typically think of compassion as a warm and friendly feeling, however, compassion is also an inner experience as it is a loving and courageous presence and a powerful resource that affects our physiology and biochemistry. Research on "The Physiological and Psychological Effects of Compassion and Anger,"[20] found that sincere, heart-focused feelings boosted the immune system whereas negative emotions could suppress the immune response nearly six hours after the emotional experience. In the book, *Buddha's Brain*, neuroscience supports that the practice of cultivating compassion is actively working in one's brain, helping to strengthen the circuitry in the regions of the anterior cingulated cortex and insula.[21(p.155)] This body of knowledge confirms that we can effect positive change in our lives, in our relationships, and in our health; it supports that it is healthy for us to practice living from the unconditional goodness of our hearts, showing genuine concern and kindness for others as well as for ourselves. The mindful practice and presence of kindness can become automatic and will naturally and subtly weave into our thoughts, actions, voices, and into our being. It is important for us to pay attention to what is happening within our bodies during conversations, observations, and interactions. The ability to differentiate between the thoughts and feelings that emerge in our internal environment with respect to the thoughts, feelings, and actions of others in our external environment will support our ability to practice empathy and compassion and help us establish and maintain healthy and respectable boundaries with our relationships.

It is important that we recognize our definition or interpretation of words as they translate into our feelings. This is essential to our ability to cultivate compassion, to forgive, heal, and transform our lives. The familiar language and conditioned beliefs around sensitivity and vulnerability may feel emotionally or mentally disruptive and "charged," or provoke a perceived sense of volatility. The internal sense of vastness and raw openness may have us feeling fragile and uneasy, even somewhat anxious because of our prior experiences and expectations. However, when we choose to explore this precious space of sensitivity and vulnerability, we begin to consider another possibility; a shift in our prior working definition emerges.

We are awakened to an awareness of a subtle unveiling and realization of sensitivity and vulnerability in their purest essence as a powerful platform where we can rest and restore... and become acutely aware of our relationships to people, external situations and events, and how they affect us or move us internally. This awareness actually serves as a *field of awareness,* our heart field expanding its outreach and influence. The heart field establishes a kind of sacred boundary that has intelligent "feelers" tuned in to both our inner and outer world. It is in and through this space we are able to gauge what is happening in both worlds simultaneously. It is through the mindful and intentional practice of accessing this profound field of knowledge and awareness that we are able to authentically engage in heartfelt communication, and make choices and decisions from acknowledging and honoring what is true and meaningful in our lives.

Healthcare is the ideal environment to cultivate a thriving emotional culture of compassion by demonstrating genuine concern for one another. The direct and rippling effects help create a positive and healing atmosphere, elevate moods, influence staff engagement and morale, and positively affect patient satisfaction and outcomes. A caring and compassionate environment is palpable by those who are within the space filled with love and concern. This type of healthy, healing conditioning benefits all persons and can help sustain efforts towards the best outcomes possible.

"I have just three things to teach: simplicity,
patience, compassion. These three are your
greatest treasures."

~ Lao Tzu

Examining Your Perceptions and Belief Systems

To make an honest assessment of what we truly desire in our lives and how we live our lives requires an open heart and objectivity without the criticism or judgment. I was inspired to identify simple yet meaningful references that would be reflective of the thoughts being conveyed in this writing. Scripture references[22] mentioned may offer you added assistance and support. You may find these references applicable in other Bible versions.

- *How many of you have prayed or are currently praying for a miracle in your personal life or for the life of a family member, friend, coworker, etc.?... a miracle that would save a life, restore your health, your relationships, your finances, and even your ability to hope and dream again.*

It can be devastating when you feel your prayers aren't getting answered. Could it be there are inconsistencies with your thoughts, mixing faith and fear, hope and doubt (James 1:5–8)? It is important to have this level of awareness about yourself and your intentions.

- *Do you have an expectation about how miracles occur?*
- *Do you have an expectation around the miracle you pray for?*
- *In what form or manner are you expecting to receive your miracle or have your miracle revealed?*

These are important questions that help you to identify your thoughts and perceptions of your prayers, heart's request, and the subsequent behavior that follows. Responses to your prayers present or reveal themselves in a variety ways.

- *Are you paying attention?*
- *Are you receptive?*
- *Are you open?*
- *Are you listening, watching, or reading... on the lookout for answers or are you closed off because of fear, doubt, or ignorance?*

As you pray for a miracle, the strength and purity of your faith matters (Hebrews 11:1-3; Mathew 17:20; Mark 11:22-24). The practice of prayer and the subsequent act of receiving an answer to a prayer is an active process (James 2:17, 2:24, and 2:26). The process of receiving a miracle requires the openness of all your available senses, which allow the spirit of absolute Faith to guide you so that your miracle can be revealed (James 5:15).

It is important to recognize that when you desire a miracle in your life, this desire is not just a feeling; it is an active, ongoing process that stems from deep within your heart. The first part of this process involves forgiveness...forgiveness of self and forgiveness of those who have hurt or wronged you (Mathew 6:14-15; Mark 11:25-26). It is a choice you make daily to harbor feelings of guilt, regret, hurt, anger, and hate. By choosing to continue hosting these negative emotions, emotions that are parasitic in nature, your ability to find peace and healing is greatly diminished. These negative emotions feast on your heart, soul, and spirit, and stifle your personal growth and healing responses. Practicing being kind, sincere, and conscious with your thoughts and actions towards yourself and others, along with keeping a heart full of faith and hope, can renew your mind, body, and spirit (Romans 5:1-2; Hebrews 10:22-25). Dismiss attempts to worry (Mathew

6:25–27, 6:33–34). Recognize that your emotions affect every aspect of your being as well as the foundation of your structural makeup . . . your cells. Feelings of joy, happiness, and enthusiasm are positively stimulating, invigorating and life enhancing; beneficial to your well-being. In contrast, the lack of luster, lack of desire, or lack of will allows for the slowing down or stagnation of cellular activity, affecting your enthusiasm and energy to support life.

Life is a journey full of many teachings and, therefore, many lessons to be learned! These lessons may be subtle or profoundly apparent. They can be found in triumphant or hardship experiences and, many times, disguised in adversities or challenges. There is a lesson or two in every adversity or challenge you face throughout your life. These lessons help you to delve deep into your core, to help you discover your strengths and weaknesses. Many times there is a message that something needs to change, to improve, to be released, to build on . . . the message calls on you to reflect on your habits, perceptions, experiences, thoughts, actions, inactions, attitude, etc. The acquired knowledge, self-discovery, and personal growth gained from perseverance and struggle enable you to define and refine your core beliefs, values, and self-worth (Romans 5:3–5; Ephesians 2:4–10; Hebrews 12:1–13; James 1:2–4).

Challenges and Adversities help you to build on your knowledge of life and of Self by drawing you closer to your Creator (Isaiah 40:29–31; Psalm 27:1; 1Peter 1:13–16; 1 Thessalonians 5:16–18). These experiences help you to recognize and connect with your spiritual self and assist you in developing the kind of wisdom that allows you to transcend to a heightened sense of awareness and fortitude; an awareness of having great purpose and abilities beyond the physical and emotional self-limiting beliefs . . . a spiritual reckoning and awakening to a journey we are all on together. Recognition, realization, and appreciation of your spiritual "being," and being fully equipped with a loving, intuitive guide, can lift personal barriers to healing (1Corinthians 2:10-16, 3:16). By accepting and applying this knowledge, you can tap into enlightenment and transformation, from which true inner peace, purpose, and power emerge (Romans 12:2). Let us openly accept and embrace the realization of the energy and love that connects people and a universe together (Hebrews 12:14-15). Know that you are not alone on this journey (Psalms 23:3-4). Allow God's love and teachings to comfort your heart and soothe your soul. Seek wisdom through His teachings so that you may be equipped with the proper tools and support necessary for a joyous, purposeful, and productive life (Ephesians 6:10-18). Together, let us pray for that miracle!

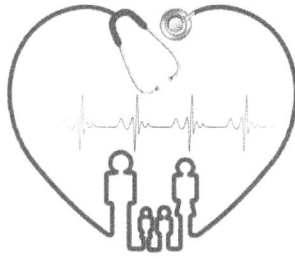

CHAPTER 8

MIND-BODY AND HEARTFUL LIVING

THE EXCHANGE

In every aspect of life, directly or indirectly, we all affect each other. Every interaction is an exchange—an interaction that involves giving and receiving... a lesson, an idea, an offering of insight, revelation, inspiration, or a heartfelt exchange of compassion and gratitude.

Restoring Hope and Possibility

My foundational training in physical therapy school taught me the value of touch. The kind of touch that was thoughtful, skillful, and conducive to healing. I also learned the value of mindfulness, which was facilitated through an awareness and subtlety of breath, movement, touch, and presence. As a student physical therapist, I had a wonderful learning experience, which significantly influenced my career and my life. I was assigned to work with a patient who had been receiving outpatient physical therapy after a serious car accident that occurred six months or so prior to my meeting her. She had sustained a major head injury, broken her pelvis, and had a few other musculoskeletal problems. When she was first injured, the priority was to get her medically stabilized and address any life threatening concerns which included a full neurological work-up.

Her physical therapy plan of care had included teaching her how to walk and to maximize her functional mobility. Pain was one of her biggest complaints during all these months. After working with her for a few visits, I recognized that pain was interfering with her quality of life and she seemed somewhat depressed and not satisfied with the gains she was making. It was troubling for me to see her this way visit after visit so I decided to talk with her in-depth about what she had been through that she could remember, and what her personal goals were for her time in therapy. She told me about how grateful she was for her life being saved and all the care she had received, however, she cried as she complained that it seemed that no one was listening to her complaints, that they did not really matter because the main focus was to help her to walk and strengthen her muscles. She cried as she further shared with me her feelings about the constant pain she would have any time she moved and the pain was especially severe when she was sitting. She spoke of her pelvis being broken which was left to heal on its own and felt it was the reason for her pain that had not yet been given any attention. Her primary mobility was the wheelchair and her desire was to be able to sit without pain. At that point of our conversation, I realized it was necessary to address her pain more directly. I received approval to add this specific area of pain management to her plan of care. I worked with her for the remaining time I had left for my training.

The day came, when my patient came in for her therapy session and began to cry, this time it was for finally having some relief. She expressed how grateful she was for me to take time to listen to her, take measures to help her identify the source of her pain, and reduce it so she could sit. She was now able to tolerate sitting, which enabled her to do homework for the college classes she planned on attending. She was now smiling and very happy.

This experience was so significant and meaningful for both of us. It radically changed the quality of her life and profoundly impacted my perspective on how to listen and care for my patients. She touched my life in such a way beyond what words can really describe. This early experience as a student forever impacted my life. It has served as a template for the kind of service I provide to this day. On our last visit together, she had a letter for me, a letter she typed while sitting. Just writing this fills my heart and brings tears to my eyes knowing what that meant for her to be able to do. I cherish this letter as it is a regular reminder for me to keep in mind why I do what I do…to make sure I listen and to care for what matters most to my patients.

Here is the letter which sits in a frame on my office shelf:

Dear Debbie,

I could write a ten page letter on how gratiful I am to you, But in the end all it would say is THANK YOU, THANKYOU AND MORE THANK YOU. Instead I am sending you my favorite blessing. I only send it to people who have touched my life in a very special way. You are one of those people, and I have truly been blessed meeting you. I wish you love and luck, in all that you do, where ever it is you may be. You'll be a great therapist. Peace to you always.......

MAY THE ROAD, RISE TO MEET YOU

MAY THE WIND, BE ALWAYS AT YOUR BACK,

MAY THE SUNSHINE WARM YOUR FACE, AND

THE RAINS FALL SOFT, UPON YOUR FIELDS.

AND UNTIL WE MEET AGAIN, MAY GOD HOLD YOU GENTLY

IN THE PALM, OF HIS HAND.

Good Luck

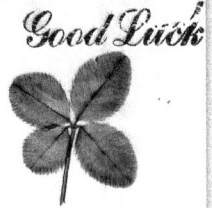

Enclosed is a four leaf clover. Take it and remember me, for I will never forget you.........

Love,

INSPIRING PEACE AND HARMONY
Inspiring Peace and Harmony

The heart responds to our experiences of the world. HeartMath® Institute has been conducting research on heart intelligence and heart-brain communication[1] providing us scientific evidence on how we can inspire peace and harmony. Their studies explore the effects of the heart's intuitive guidance on human behavior and in building social coherence which can help us deepen our connection to self and others. Neuro-cardiology research[1] has identified that the heart has an intrinsic nervous system that acts like a brain, however functions independently from the brain and links to every major organ in the body sending information throughout the body to keep it working in harmony.

The heart and brain are in continuous dialogue. Research has identified that the heart communicates to the brain through the nervous system, pulse waves, hormones and neurotransmitters, and electromagnetic fields.[1] Such heart influences on the brain centers are involved in our emotional experiences, perceptions, and cognitive performance.

The heart is a powerful electromagnetic generator able to generate an electromagnetic field that can be detected several feet away from the body.[2] This means that we have the potential to be in each others' field every day. Research at the Institute of Heartmath® showed that information pertaining to a person's emotional state is communicated through the body via the heart's electromagnetic field.[2]

We are accustomed to hearing about cortisol and adrenalin, hormones which serve us well during stress and crisis situations. There is also a hormone called oxytocin which plays as the counterpart to these stress response hormones. The natural flow and balance of these hormones are essential to our health and well-being, and significantly contribute to our perspective of humanity and life as a whole. More and more is being discussed and researched about the hormone oxytocin. When it is released it supports the bonding of babies with their mothers as it is the hormone of trust and connection. Oxytocin is released through mother's milk, orgasm, feelings of unconditional love and appreciation, and authentic heart to heart connections. This hormone opens us to explore relationships, and encourages intimacy and collaboration. With consistent practice, we can intentionally produce more oxytocin through our breathing of love and compassion for ourselves and others. Oxytocin can be produced "on demand" without force or effort, for the production and flow of this biochemical love potion can be generated through sincere, heartfelt appreciation and acts of kindness. We can actually learn to calm and reorganize our stressed and burdened nervous system and positively influence our heart rhythm patterns with the facilitation of oxytocin release inspiring peace and harmony within. The release of oxytocin in the body can also contribute to a positive coherent emotional state that can be communicated through a person's electromagnetic field.

Our life experiences, conditioned behaviors, and emotions have an effect on our biochemistry and physiology. In neurobiological research conducted by Zak and Colleagues[3,4] on trust and trustworthiness, they identified that higher oxytocin levels were associated with trust and trustworthy behavior, and the presence of this hormone may contribute to motivating cooperation.

The most valuable gift we can give to each other is trust. Not trust in the sense that we won't make mistakes but trust that the tenderness, fragility, and vulnerability of our deepest heartfelt emotions will be honored and valued as if they were our own. We are interdependent beings all capable of giving and receiving this wonderful gift. True, authentic, and unconditional heart-to-heart connections convey without words acceptance, and have an undercurrent of love, compassion, empathy, and appreciation. This way of relating opens the door to trust and forgiveness, to hope and possibility, to a new friendship or intimate relationship. Tears may flow so that hearts may grow. We can all learn how to trust, allow ourselves to access and embody a true sense and state of trust with desired intention and practice.

"Teach this triple truth to all: A generous heart, kind speech, and a life of service and compassion are the things which renew humanity."

~ Buddha

THE HEART OF MINDFULNESS AND INTENTION

- *Are you genuinely interested and engaged throughout your day or are you trying to get through your day, running on autopilot?*

Finding ways to integrate your life into a work life "balance" is about the interplay. It is about being mindful and inviting meaningful moments into your life. From this approach to your day, you are more aware, engaged, enthusiastic and energized as your creativity is sparked and inspiration naturally happens. Mindfulness can help you focus, make decisions, improve interpersonal relationships, improve performance, and effectively deal with uncertainty. Mindfulness also helps you to appreciate yourself, others, and situations for the lessons or insights that may accompany the experience, instead of possible drama or judgment that could present itself just as easily without this practice. Mindfulness helps you listen more deeply and dissolve expectations, realizing that there is no true right or wrong scenario, or a positive or negative outcome.[5] Mindfulness is about noticing, witnessing, unlocking, taking the brake off, and taking a breath as you open to all of life experiences as they are… Living with the illusion of control grips you in fear and can stifle you, being disabling at times when the mindful practice helps you to remember there is an opportunity here and now to learn something new, to grow, and to let go.

Mindfulness opens you to a wider lens of perspective which may have its challenges and opportunities. Being mindful about your abilities, inabilities, feelings, and outlook allows you to be authentically present and accepting of yourself and your life, not needing to have all the answers. You become grounded, more transparent, and conscious with the practice of mindfulness. You learn to simply and profoundly be present, feeling more life flow through your body, as you are being ever more connected with life all around you. Mindfulness helps you to have focused attention but not be so laser focused that you miss something important or potentially dangerous happening around you.

Mindfulness is a powerful, yet simple, quiet, reflective, contemplative practice that cultivates sensitivity and flexibility. It is a waking practice that has personally brought greater meaning and inspiration into my life. It has been a helpful resource to keep me together and grounded, has kept my mind sound and heart open amidst the pressures, demands, and grief I have recently experienced. Mindfulness can be brought into any situation, anywhere, and at any time.

SELF-LEADERSHIP
Reframe Your View

Vitality, Exhilaration, and Joy are energizing and stimulating to the human spirit, yet few truly live with this heightened level of emotion and enthusiasm. I have a personal philosophy for my life: to be a positive influence wherever I go. It is always my intention to be of goodwill, to inspire, and to motivate anyone and everyone that enters my sphere of influence.

When working with people that want or need your service, offering a smile will visually and energetically send out an uplifting message that you care. Wherever I am, I observe the people around me. I notice people who work hard but have complacent attitudes. Many complain, but do nothing to change themselves or the situation. It's easier to go with the flow than to create your own flow. Many people make numerous excuses for their situations. I have done so myself.

- *How easy is it to get caught up in the whirlwind of life events and even feel stuck at times?*
- *How easy is it to forget the privilege you have to be able to choose your perspective?*

It's time to start paying closer attention to your thoughts, feelings, and behaviors.

- *How often are you holding your breath throughout the day?*
- *Are you a reactor or a responder?*

Practice objectivity; step outside yourself and become the observer. Remember your language and intentions matter. "Isn't that interesting?"

- *Are you really committed to being successful in life and in your business?*

When you are truly committed to success, there are no obstacles too great to overcome. There's no settling or complaining. When you have the WILL, you'll FIND or MAKE a way!

Envision the Change and Progress You Desire

We've all heard that if you keep on doing what you've been doing, you'll keep on getting what you've been getting. Many of us can talk a great talk but there is no consistency or purposeful action to the talk; we are in the TRY mode (perpetual motion like a hamster on a wheel), and the WHY mode (why aren't things working out the way I want them to?). We must commit to self-discipline, to developing habits that get us desired results. It's time for LESS TALK and MORE ACTION. Put your energy and attention on purposeful, productive activity designed on get-ting results. Identify each aspect of your life— health, finances, family, social, relationships, etc. Write them down. Make the connection . . . Visualize and Feel the emotion of achieving the results you desire. Determine action-oriented goals for each; com-mit to what you will do to work towards making your vision a reality.

Inner Honor Code

Honor yourself and your life by holding yourself to a way of being and living that you will not violate nor will you allow anyone else to violate. This puts full responsibility on you to be mindful, present, and committed to your growth, your success, your happiness.

- *Are your emotions triggered or body senses heightened by some-one's comment, a look, a sound, a similar experience?*

Keep in mind, people, situations and circumstances reflect for us things we may still need to work on, emotions not fully pro-cessed or dealt with. In these moments when your emotions are feeling reactive, there may be a tendency to lash out, blame, or possibly exhibit aggressive or violent behaviors, moving the atten-tion away from yourself looking to the outside world as being responsible for disrupting your life, making you feel the way you feel. This outward display is an avoidance behavior that will continue to show up until you take full responsibility for any emotion that rises in you based on what has been said, done, acted on, etc. In these very sensitive and volatile moments, you have to pause and realize that what is being stirred in you, what is being revealed in you is for your own good, your own awakening, and ultimately for you to address and resolve. This pause gives you a moment to breathe and turn inward to quietly tune in and connect and reflect. An expression of gratitude through your breathing, through your voice and through your heart can go a long way to assist you in this vulnerable state. This is a practice you must choose to partake in. You have survival instincts that are your default pattern, just remember you have the ability to choose.

- *Are you ready to thrive, to live freely, to experience love and life fully, to be in the presence of glory, grace, and gratitude?*

Make time for yourself…quiet time; inspiring breaths which support wisdom, mindfulness, love, and appreciation.

"We must be the change
we wish to see in the world."

~ Gandhi

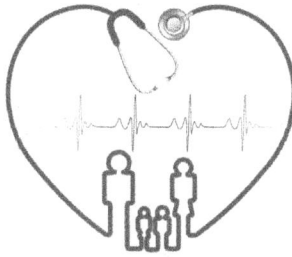

SOURCES

PREFACE: THE BUSINESS OF LIVING WELL THROUGH SELF-CARE MANAGEMENT

1. Abramson S, Stein J, Schaufele M, Frates E, Rogan S. Personal exercise habits and counseling practices of primary care physicians: a national survey. *Clin J Sport Med*. 2000;10(1):40-8.

2. Better self-management improves outcomes for chronic pain care. American Pain Society Web site. http://americanpainsociety.org/about-us/press-room/better-self-management-improves-outcomes-for-chronic-pain-care. Published 2016. Accessed Sept. 5, 2016.

CHAPTER 1: ACT ON YOUR HEALTH

1. Leading Causes of Death. Center for Disease Control and Prevention Web site. http://www.cdc.gov/nchs/fastats/leading-causes-of-death.htm. Updated March 17, 2017. Accessed February 22, 2018.

2. Chronic Disease Overview. Center for Disease Control and Prevention Web site. http://www.cdc.gov/chronicdisease/overview/index.htm. Updated June 28, 2017. Accessed February 22, 2018.

3. American Heart Association Recommendations for Physical Activity in Adults. American Heart Association Web site. http://www.heart.org/HEARTORG/HealthyLiving/PhysicalActivity/FitnessBasics/American-Heart-Association-Recommendations-for-Physical-Activity-in-Adults_UCM_307976_Article.jsp#.WA-_e_krKM8. Updated July 27, 2016. Accessed October 25, 2016.
4. Jensen GM, Mostrom E. *Handbook of Teaching and Learning for Physical Therapists.* 3rd ed. St. Louis, MO:Butterworth Heinemann; 2013.

CHAPTER 2: LEADING HEALTH INDICATORS

1. About Healthy People 2020. Healthy People Web site. https://www.healthypeople.gov/2020/About-Healthy-People. Updated October 27, 2016. Accessed September 3, 2016.
2. 2020 Topics and Objectives. Healthy People Web site. https://www.healthypeople.gov/2020/topics-objectives. Updated October 27, 2016. Accessed September 3, 2016
3. Leading Health Indicators. Healthy People Web site. https://www.healthypeople.gov/2020/Leading-Health-Indicators. Updated October 27, 2016. Accessed September 3, 2016.
4. Healthy People 2020 Leading Health Indicators: Progress Update. Healthy People Web site. https://www.healthypeople.gov/2020/leading-health-indicators/Healthy-People-2020-Leading-Health-Indicators%3A-Progress-Update. Updated October 27, 2016. Accessed Sept. 3, 2016.
5. Cooperberg MR, Birkmeyer JD, Litwin MS. Defining high quality health care. *Urol Oncol.* 2009;27(4):411-6.
6. Berkowitz L. Defining healthcare innovation. *Clinical*

Innovation + Technology. June 25, 2103. http://www.clinical-innovation.com/topics/clinical-practice/defining-healthcare-innovation. Accessed September 3, 2016.

7. Abramson S, Stein J, Schaufele M, Frates E, Rogan S. Personal exercise habits and counseling practices of primary care physicians: a national survey. *Clin J Sport Med.* 2000;10(1):40-8.

8. Physical Activity. Healthy People Web site. https://www.healthypeople.gov/2020/data-search/Search-the-Data#objid=5056. Updated October 27, 2016. Accessed September 3, 2016.

9. Walk with a Doc Web site. http://walkwithadoc.org/. Accessed September 3, 2016.

10. Exercise is Medicine Web site http://www.exerciseismedicine.org/. Accessed September 3, 2016.

11. Greenwood JL, Joy EA, Stanford J. The physical activity vital sign: a primary care tool to guide counseling for obesity. *J Phys Act Health.* 2010;7(5):571-6.

12. Coleman KJ, Ngor E, Reynolds K, et al. Initial validation of an exercise "vital sign" in electronic medical records. *Med Sci Sports Exerc.* 2012;44(11):2071-6.

13. Kountz DS. Strategies for improving low health literacy. *Postgrad Med.* 2009;121(5):171-7.

CHAPTER 3: THE ROAD AHEAD

1. Boutayeb A, Boutayeb S. The burden of non communicable diseases in developing countries. *International Journal for Equity in Health.* 2005;4:2. doi:10.1186/1475-9276-4-2.

2. Phillips E, Pojednic R, Polak R, Bush J, Trilk J. Including lifestyle medicine in undergraduate medical curricula. *Med Educ Online.* 2015;20:26150. http://dx.doi.org/10.3402/meo.v20.26150.

3. Lifestyle Medicine Education Collaborative Web site. http://lifestylemedicineeducation.org/. Accessed September 3, 2016.

4. Landsman-Dijkstra JJ, van Wijck R, Groothoff JW. The long-term lasting effectiveness on self-efficacy, attribution style, expression of emotions and quality of life of a body awareness program for chronic a-specific psychosomatic symptoms. *Patient Educ Couns.* 2006;60(1):66-79.

5. Kripalani S, Jacobson TA, Mugalla IC, et al. Health literacy and the quality of physician-patient communication during hospitalization. *J Hosp Med.* 2010;5(5):269-75.

6. Wynia MK, Osborn CY. Health literacy and communication quality in health care organizations. *J Health Commun.* 2010;15(Suppl 2):102–115.

7. Wallace LS, Rogers ES, Roskos SE, et al. Brief report: screening Items to identify patients with limited health literacy skills. *J Gen Intern Med.* 2006;21(8):874–877.

8. Chew LD, Griffin JM, Partin MR, et al. Validation of screening questions for limited health literacy in a large VA outpatient population. *J Gen Intern Med.* 2008;23(5):561–566.

9. Dwamena F, Holmes-Rovner M, Gaulden CM, et al. Interventions for providers to promote a patient-centred approach in clinical consultations. *Cochrane Database Syst Rev.* 2012;12.

10. Exercise is Medicine Web site. http://www.exerciseismedicine.org/. Accessed September 3, 2016.

11. Shapiro SL, Schwartz GE, Bonner G. Effects of mindfulness-based stress reduction on medical and premedical students. *J Behav Med.* 1998;21:581-599.

12. Friese M, Messner C, Schaffner Y. Mindfulness meditation counteracts self-control depletion. *Conscious Cogn.* 2012;21:1016-1022.

13. Shapiro SL, Carlson LE, Astin JA, Freedman B. Mechanisms of mindfulness. J *Clin Psychol.* 2006;62:373-386.
14. Zeidan F, Johnson SK, Diamond BJ, David Z, Goolkasian P. Mindfulness meditation improves cognition: Evidence of brief mental training. *Conscious Cogn.* 2010;19(2):597-605.
15. Zeidan F, Gordon N, Merchant J, Goolkasian P. The effects of brief mindfulness meditation training on experimentally induced pain. *J Pain.* 2010;11(3):199-209.
16. Tang Y, Ma Y, Wang J, et al. Short-term meditation training improves attention and self-regulation. *Proceed Nat Acad Sci.* 2007;104;17152-17156.
17. Taylor DG, Mireault, GC. Mindfulness self-regulation: a comparison of long-term to short-term meditators. *J Transpers Psychol.* 2008;40(1):88-99.
18. Majumdar M, Grossman P, Dietz-Waschkowski B, Kersig S, Walach H. Does mindfulness meditation contribute to health? Outcome evaluation of German sample. *J Alt Comple Med.* 2002;8(6):719-730.
19. Kabat-Zinn J. Mindfulness-based interventions in context: past, present, and future. *Clin Psychol Sci Prac.* 2003;10:144-156.
20. Holzel BK, Lazar SW, Gard T, Schuman-Olivier Z, Vago DR, Ott U. How does mindfulness meditation work? Proposing mechanisms of action from a conceptual and neural perspective. *Perspec on Psychol Sci.* 2011;6(6):537-559.
21. Kabat-Zinn J. An outpatient program in behavioral medicine for chronic pain patients based on the practice of mindfulness meditation: theoretical considerations and preliminary results. *Gen Hosp Psychiatry.*1982;4:33-47.
22. Robins CJ, Keng SL, Ekblad AG, Brantley JG. Effects of mindfulness-based stress reduction on emotional experience and expression: a randomized controlled trial. *J. Clin Psychol.* 2012;68(1):117-131.

CHAPTER 4: PERSPECTIVES MATTER

1. Hill N. *Think and Grow Rich*. Greenwich, CT:Fawcett Publications;1960.

CHAPTER 5: INFLUENCES ON HEALTH AND WELL-BEING

1. Blanding M. Workplace stress responsible for up to $190B in annual U.S. healthcare costs. *Forbes*. January 26, 2015. http://onforb.es/1CrYbzp. Accessed September 3, 2016.

2. Lynch S. Why your workplace might be killing you: Stanford scholars identify 10 work stressors that are destroying your health. *Stanford Business*. February 23, 2015. https://www.gsb.stanford.edu/insights/why-your-workplace-might-be-killing-you. Accessed September 3, 2016.

3. Health Advocate. Stress in the workplace meeting the challenge. http://healthadvocate.com/downloads/webinars/stress-workplace.pdf. Accessed September 3, 2016.

4. Chemtob, CM, Novaco, RW, Hamada, RS, Gross, DM, Smith, G. Anger regulation deficits in combat-related posttraumatic stress disorder. *J Trauma Stress*. 1997;10(1):17-36.

5. Taft CT, Niles BL. Assessment and treatment of anger in combat-related PTSD. http://www.humana-military.com/library/pdf/assessment-treatment-anger-combat-related-ptsd.pdf. Accessed September 23, 2016

6. Compassion Fatigue. The American Institute of Stress Web site. www.stress.org/military/for-practitionersleaders/compassion-fatigue/. Accessed September 17, 2016.

7. Newell JM, MacNeil GA. Professional burnout, vicarious trauma, secondary traumatic stress, and compassion fatigue: A review of theoretical terms, risk factors, and preventive methods for clinicians and researchers. *Best Practices in Mental Health*. 2010;6(2):57-68.

8. Seppala E, Cameron K. Proof that positive work cultures are more productive. *Harvard Business Review*. December 1, 2015. https://hbr.org/2015/12/proof-that-positive-work-cultures-are-more-productive. Accessed 9/17/16.

CHAPTER 6: INTRINSIC INFLUENCES ON CHANGE

1. Jensen GM, Mostrom E. *Handbook of Teaching and Learning for Physical Therapists*. 3rd ed. St. Louis, MO:Butterworth-Heinemann;2013.
2. Orji R, Vassileva J, Mandryk R. Towards an effective health interventions design: an extension of the health belief model. *Online J Public Health Inform*. 2012; 4(3):e9. doi: 10.5210/ojphi.v4i3.4321.
3. Rollnick S, Miller WR, Butler CC. *Motivational Interviewing in Health Care: Helping Patients Change Behavior*. New York, NY:Guilford Press;2008.

CHAPTER 7: SELF-CARE MANAGEMENT

1. American Heart Association. Heart disease and stroke statistics—2012 update. *Circulation*. 2012;125(1):e2-e220. doi:10.1161/CIR.0b013e31823ac046.
2. Lloyd-Jones DM, Leip EP, Larson MG, et al. Prediction of lifetime risk for cardiovascular disease by risk factor burden at 50 years of age. *Circulation*. 2006;113:791-798.
3. Greaves CJ, Campbell JL. Supporting self-care in general practice. *Brit J Gen Prac*. 2007; 57: 814-821.
4. Ory MG, Smith ML, Ahn S, Jiang L, Lorig K, Whitelaw N. National study of chronic disease self-management: Age comparison of outcome findings. *Health Educ Behav*. 2014;41(1)34-42.
5. Chronic Disease Self-Management Facts. National Council on Aging Website: http://www.ncoa.org/press-room/

fact-sheets/chronic-disease.html. Accessed 10/28/16.

6. Lorig KR, Sobel D, Ritter PL, Hobbs M, Laurent D. Effect of a self-management program on patients with chronic disease. *Eff Clin Pract.* 2001;4:256-262.

7. Ahn S, Basu R, Smith ML, Jiang L, Lorig K, Whitelaw N, Ory MG. The impact of chronic disease self-management programs: Healthcare savings through a community-based intervention. *BMC Pub Health.* 2013;13(1):1141.

8. Ory MG, Ahn S, Jiang L, Lorig K, Ritter P, Laurent DL, Whitelaw N, Smith ML. National study of chronic disease self-management: Six month outcome findings. *J Aging Health.* 2013;25:1258.

9. Sobel DS, Lorig KR, Hobbs M. Chronic condition self-management program: from development to dissemination. *Perm J.* 2002;6(2):11-8.

10. Chronic Disease Self-Management Program. Stanford Medicine Patient Education Website. http://patienteducation. stanford.edu/programs/cdsmp.html. Accessed October 25, 2016.

11. Bayliss EA, Ellis JL, Steiner JF. Barriers to self-management and quality-of-life outcomes in seniors with multimorbidities. *Ann Fam Med.* 2007; 5:395-402.

12. Bandura A. The primacy of self-regulation in health promotion. *Applied Psychol.* 2005;54(2):245-254.

13. Bandura A. Perceived self-efficacy in cognitive development and functioning. *Educ Psychologist.* 1993;28(2):117-148.

14. Bandura A. Health promotion by social cognitive means. *Health Educ Behav.* 2004;31(2):143-164.

15. Maibach E, Murphy DA. Self-efficacy in health promotion research and practice: conceptualization and measurement. *Health Educ Research.* 1995;10(1):37-50.

16. Sousa ZAA, Silva JG, Ferreira MA. Knowledge and practices of teenagers about health: Implications for the

lifestyle and self care. *Escola Anna Nery.* 2014;*18*(3): 400-406.

17. Modi AC, Pai AL, Hommel KA, et al. Pediatric self-management: A framework for research, practice, and policy. *Pediatrics.* 2012; 129: e473-e485.

18. Sawin KJ, Bellin MH, Roux G, Buran CF, Brei TJ. The experience of self-management in adolescent women with spina bifida. *Rehab Nursing.* 2009;34(1):26-38.

19. Helgeson VS, Reynolds KA, Siminerio L, Escobar O, Becker D. Parent and adolescent distribution of responsibility for diabetes self-care: Links to health outcomes. *J Pediatr Psychol.* 2008;33(5):497–508.

20. Rein G, Atkinson M, McCraty R. The Physiological and psychological effects of compassion and anger. *J Advance Med.* 1995; 8 (2): 87-105.

21. Hanson R. *Buddha's Brain: The Practical Neuroscience of Happiness, Love & wisdom.* Oakland, CA: New Harbinger Publications;2009.

22. Ryrie CC. *The Ryrie Study Bible: New International Version.* Grand Rapids, MI: Zondervan Publishing; 1994.

CHAPTER 8: MIND-BODY AND HEARTFUL LIVING

1. Heart-Brain Communication. HeartMath Institute Web site. https://www.heartmath.org/research/science-of-the-heart/heart-brain-communication/. Accessed September 3, 2016.

2. Energetic Communication. HeartMath Institute Web site. https://www.heartmath.org/research/science-of-the-heart/energetic-communication/. Accessed September 3, 2106.

3. Zak PJ, Kurzban R, Matzner WT. The neurobiology of trust. *Ann N Y Acad Sci.* 2004;1032:224-227.

4. Zak PJ, Kurzban R, Matzner WT Oxytocin is associated with human trustworthiness. *Horm Behav.* 2005;48(5):522-527.

5. Harvard Business Review. Mindfulness in the age of complexity. *Harvard Business Review*. March 2014. https://hbr.org/2014/03/mindfulness-in-the-age-of-complexity. Accessed September 3, 2016.

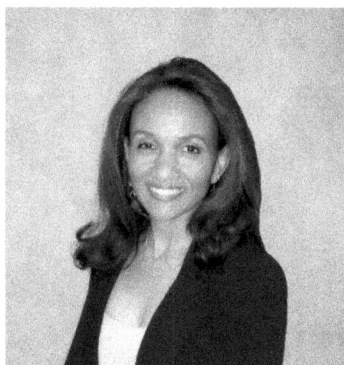

Dr. Deborah Howell is a health and life transition coach committed to cultivating and promoting the well-being of health professionals experiencing overcare and compassion fatigue. Through heart-focused retreats and training termed, "Rehab for the Heart," health professionals and executives re-charge, renew, and restore PASSION, COMPASSION, HEALTH, and VITALITY for living life inspired with greater joy and fulfillment. Dr. Howell's Rehab for the Heart is rooted in Emotional Muscle Fitness® – a practical and integrative methodology that enhances the ability to effectively manage stress, cope with change, and build emotional capacity and resilience.

Self-Care for Health Professionals and Executives
www.healthcarerebootcamp.com

CONNECT on Facebook!
Facebook.com/selfcareinhealthcare

www.ingramcontent.com/pod-product-compliance
Lightning Source LLC
Chambersburg PA
CBHW072012290326
41934CB00007BA/1066